Shoulder Surgery Recovery

Over 100 Tips and Strategies to Make It Much Easier

by

Anne Talmage Cooksey

TABLE OF CONTENTS

Dedicated with much love to my husband, John. Every day I spend with you is a blessing and a bonus.

INTRODUCTION

I was drained. It had been an exhausting day. I had washed six loads of smelly camp clothes in the hotel laundry, been yelled at by a scary woman with issues and had a happy, teary reunion with my family. I wanted a hot shower. I stripped off my clothes, pulled back the shower curtain and stepped into the tub. As soon as my feet touched the slick enamel, they slid out from under me to the left and I was airborne. My head pinballed around the tub and my right shoulder slammed into the side. Next thing I knew I was sitting in the tub facing the faucet thinking, "What the hell?" and "I hurt." I was afraid to move. My husband was watching television in the next room. I kept saying "help me...help me...help me…" in this creepy croak as if I said it any louder, my head might fall off. He ran in. Off to the emergency room we went…

If you're in the middle of doctor appointments contemplating shoulder surgery, you have lots to think about and lots of decisions to make. You may be an adventurous soul who wants to bring your cryo cuff on your Caribbean cruise one week after surgery. Or a daredevil like the gentleman who rode a roller coaster at Six Flags in Dallas three weeks after surgery while wearing his immobilizer sling. You may be like me, terrified of having the surgery and looking for someone, anyone, to tell you,"Nah, you're fine. You don't need it." Whichever one you are, it helps to have a plan.

Every shoulder surgery is different. Treatments and therapies vary. Stay in close consultation with your physicians and medical professionals. Each of us goes at our own pace. You might be in Phase 3 and sailing right along in your recovery. Then you pick something up too heavy, too soon, and find yourself back in Phase 1 doing pendulum swings again. You might be overly afraid or cautious and feel you are being pushed too fast through physical therapy. Finding your voice and learning to set boundaries as you learn what your body can and cannot do is a big part of recovery. Your healing is as unique as you are. What began for me as a white-knuckled ride dissolved into a lot of laughter and tears as I worked through my fears to a successful recovery on the other side.

Anyone you know who has had shoulder surgery is a good resource. Ask them every question you can think of – there are no stupid or too intrusive questions, believe me. Before surgery, it's all a deep mystery that makes you an insatiable bottomless pit -- you want to know every gory detail so you can prepare yourself. You'll also find out, after weeks or months of intense groundwork, you can't completely prepare because life likes throwing curve balls. Even putting on your underpants becomes an adventure.

Everything in this book is how I experienced my own personal shoulder surgery recovery. These tips, suggestions and products are based on my own wacky ride. You may find some products are great and some are just okay for you. Some retailers are the bomb and some make you stamp your foot. Take what you like and leave the rest. Hopefully this book will serve to blow a window open inside your brain and realize how many cool resources there are ready to help you through your own recovery. Use this stuff as a jumping off point to develop your own methods, inventions and discoveries under the guidance of your doctors and physical therapists.

Get ready for a twelve to eighteen month progression that will take you to infinity and beyond in terms of pain management, patience, baby steps, depression, exhilaration, and hopefully, a big dollop of compassion for yourself as you learn to take each day one minute at a time. This book is jam-packed with over 100 different tips, suggestions and products to help make your life after rotator cuff surgery a little easier.

Chapter 1:

DIAGNOSIS

The rotator cuff in my right shoulder had been deteriorating for some time. I'd been rear-ended in several car accidents, had a diving accident, and in 2012, fell in a hotel bathtub. My right shoulder took the brunt of the fall. That was the beginning of the end of my rotator cuff. I'd been a children's entertainer for most of my adult life and played my guitar as part of the act. After I recuperated from the neck injuries caused by the fall in that shower, I noticed my shoulder was painful after playing but I didn't pay much attention. I figured I was just getting older.

The next year we traveled as a family on a train to Canada. We took lots of baggage and I hoisted many of the bags over my head. That was really stupid. I have two strong, healthy boys and a husband who lifts weights. Why did I vote myself best equipped to organize and move the luggage around? Because I was an obsessive control freak who lifted them when no one was looking because I knew they would stop me. The last remaining strand of my rotator cuff gave up the ghost on that trip.

Now any time I practiced or played my guitar it was really hard to raise my right arm up and over the instrument. When I tried to help my friend conduct a children's program, I couldn't raise my arm up without stabbing pain. My arm ached at night. I couldn't reach to turn off my bedside lamp without extreme discomfort. I couldn't sleep cuddled up on my right side. It had gone from annoying to "twist the damn thing off and get me a new one!"

Rotator cuff muscles are the stabilizing muscles in your shoulder. These muscles allow you to reach up overhead, lift your arm up and over things like a guitar, raise your hand to ask a question, swim, throw a ball and play tennis or golf. You can have an injury after lifting something heavy or a bad fall on your shoulder. Your rotator cuff can also just wear out after years and years of use. When your arm aches at night, even waking you up out of a sound sleep, and you have weakness or are unable to raise your arm, most likely it's your rotator cuff. When you go into your doctor's office, they will examine your arm to determine how much weakness is present. X-rays or an MRI are scheduled next.

After three months of taking ibuprofen for the pain, I ended up at my doctor's office because I thought I had an ulcer due to all the OTC anti-inflammatory drugs I was taking. "Why are you taking all this ibuprofen?" "Because my arm hurts all the time and it's not getting better!" She sent me for x-rays, then an MRI. The MRI hurt like fire. I asked the technician if that was normal and he said, "yes, if you have a really big tear." Turns out I had a massive full thickness tear of the supraspinatus in my right rotator cuff. Great. I didn't have time to deal with a crappy arm. I had too much other stuff going on in my life: my husband was recovering and getting back in remission from a rare disease, I was running two businesses with my husband, plus homeschooling my two boys. I ended up back in my doctor's office, sobbing and using up all her tissues. It was time to take care of myself and get my arm fixed.

I went to the recommended orthopedic surgeon to discover my options. She was impersonal, clinical and succinct. She said my shoulder was completely frozen and I was not a candidate for physical therapy or cortisone shots. I also needed to make a decision to have shoulder surgery right away or I would gradually lose the use of my arm and could look forward to a life of pain, degenerative arthritis and deterioration. Ouch!

If you're uncomfortable with the first opinion and you feel rushed or unsure, take a deep breath. When the first orthopedic surgeon says "jump!", you don't have to ask "how high?" You don't have to decide in ten minutes. A torn rotator cuff may hurt but it's a mechanical issue, not a life-threatening one. You need to feel comfortable and satisfied with your orthopedic surgeon. Look for one whose bedside manner you can live with and whose skill in this particular surgery is highly-rated. Get another opinion. Ask people who have had this surgery who their surgeon was and if they were pleased with the results. Spend as much time finding a good fit as you would picking out a new car. This is your shoulder, the most mobile joint in your body, we're talking about here -- take your time and find yourself the best surgeon with the most successful track record.

At my husband's suggestion, I called a friend who's a personal trainer. She raved about her orthopedic surgeon. I got his number and went for a second opinion. When he walked in to examine me, it felt like sunshine had walked into the room. He went through my range of motion and said "yes, you have a frozen shoulder as well as the massive tear. Let's get it unfrozen so you don't have to deal with that pain on top of the pain after surgery. We'll give you a shot of cortisone and get you signed up for physical therapy. When you have your range of motion back and you are ready, we will repair your rotator cuff." No drama, no pressure, just common sense and a whole lot of positive thinking. This was a plan I could live with.

For twelve weeks I worked on my range of motion at physical therapy. By the end of physical therapy I could raise my arm as if to answer a question. But I couldn't get it back down without pain. I still couldn't lift my arm up and over my guitar to strum without muscle spasms or pain. That's where the supraspinatus muscle comes in. In order to put my hand down by itself or lift my arm out to the side, I would need to get that repaired. I planned to have the surgery in April, 2015.

Chapter 2:

PREPARATION

It's important to be as healthy as possible before surgery. And you can do everything you can in your power to get to that point and still miss the mark. We are human. Surgery is intimidating. Anesthesia is scary. But so is driving in your car every day. We just choose not to dwell on the "oh my God, I could die!" aspect and think about the party we're going to or the movie we can't wait to see. Elective surgery is in its own category because if you choose to, you could cancel. You could choose to live with the pain and take a pass. But you are choosing to undergo pain for a greater reward; which, by the way, is very brave. Go you!

In the meantime, you'd like to be at your physical best when the surgery happens. Back to the we are human thing and are about to do something scary by choice...right. Lots of people stress eat to soothe the beast that is crocheting your insides together with rusty needles. It wants cookies, mashed potatoes, Reese's peanut butter cups and ice cream. Don't beat yourself up. You're going through enough with all the plans and decisions you have to make. Toss it a green salad and some protein at least once a day and let it have the cookies. Obviously if you are a diabetic or have a serious health issue, then follow your doctor's instructions. But if you are just suffering from a severe case of hand to mouth disease due to nerves, let it go. Time enough to cut back when you're back out on the tennis court or doing curls in the gym with your brand-new shoulder.

You won't be able to plan for every possible situation before your surgery date, but you can do your best to run through as many scenarios in your head and prepare accordingly. There are going to be the days in Phase Two when you promise to make your kids homemade pizza (frozen crust, jarred sauce and shredded mozzarella -- you put it together, it's homemade!), but what you thought was mozzarella turns out to be shredded parmesan and you still can't drive. You give a desperate shout out to your friend whose husband drives over with two bags of mozzarella and saves the day. You cannot purchase enough cheese ahead to stave off every pizza emergency.

There are many things you can prepare ahead of your surgery date. You can plan what you're going to wear and where you're going to sleep. You can research and purchase the vitamins, supplements and over-the-counter medications you want to have at hand. You can figure out ahead of time how you are going to delegate meal preparation and who's in charge of what chores in your household. You can hire additional help. You can chart out and streamline business and school obligations for the next few months.

I was a fairly calm and reasonable person on the surface, but I was one happy thought away from a full blown anxiety attack. I was going to be in a sling for six weeks and my repair would take a full eighteen months to reach full range of motion and strength. Setting the date made it very real. It was now December 2014. I had four months to prepare. In addition to being anxious, I was obsessive-compulsive. I decided to take all my nervous energy and approach my upcoming surgery like a paramilitary operation.

I stepped up my appointments to my chiropractor to have the best range of motion and least inflammation going into surgery. Ultrasound on my shoulder was helpful to relieve ongoing inflammation. I also checked back in with my physical therapist to make sure I had not lost any range of motion. Physically, I was ready to have the repair done. Time to prepare for battle.

Household Bills

If you don't already, it's a good idea to have your household accounts organized before surgery. Not only do you need an idea of what bills get paid when on a monthly basis, but it would make your life easier if you prepaid your bills 1-2 months ahead of time right before the surgery. That may seem overboard, but if you are the chief bill payer at your house, your spouse is going to have a hard enough time taking care of you without having to remember to pay the utility bill. And if you live alone, you'll be happier having one less thing to think about during your recovery. Using a keyboard and mouse in the first few weeks is tricky, especially if surgery was done on your dominant hand's side. You can't move your arm away from your body for the first four to six weeks. You can also put the bills on automatic draft from your checking account so you aren't stressing over them. Try to get the whole shebang on autopilot for at least three to four weeks so if a crisis does happen, you can focus on it and not on a bunch of little yappy stuff.

Putting Your Business on Autopilot

If you run your own business, make sure your staff is well-briefed on what needs to be accomplished in your absence. Again, make sure all bills, tax paperwork and other daily, weekly and monthly tasks are gone over and delegated. Do it now while your brain and all other parts of your body are up and functioning. Check inventories, employee schedules, payroll and emergency procedures. Do dry runs where they have to role play situations that may arise.

Carpools and After School Help

If you have children and they attend public or private school, make sure you have carpooling and back-up drivers lined up. Schedule rides to different activities. You aren't going to be so out of it that you can't verbally help with homework, but you may need to enlist an older student for after school homework assistance for science or art projects. If you have small children, try to get some extra help to care for them during your recovery. If you don't have extra hands to help you, you may be tempted to move or lift which would put your shoulder repair in jeopardy.

Homeschooling

If you homeschool, you can prepay and line up tutors, order extra curriculum, and plan history or science DVDs to watch together as you recuperate. Purchase online teaching services, such as Teaching Textbooks, Super Teacher Worksheets and Time4Learning. Teaching Textbooks has math workbooks and CD-Roms. It offers curriculum from 3rd grade math all the way up to Pre-Calculus. It's more expensive than some, ranging from $99 for just the CD-Roms up to $190 for CD-Roms plus workbooks for the higher grades, but well worth the money. Super Teacher Worksheets is $19.95 for a year's membership for unlimited printing of worksheets including math, spelling, cursive, language arts, reading comprehension and lots more. Time4Learning is an online comprehensive service for homeschool curriculum, after school learning and skill building. It is $19.95/month per student for PreK-8th and $30/month per student for high school. If you have more than one student, the price drops to $14.95/month for each additional student. Scholastic.com offers free printable worksheets in a range of subjects as well.

Print out lesson plans and worksheets, organize schoolwork folders, print schedules and line up people to drive them to their various activities. However, in your frenzied school planning, you may hear comments like "You know she's not going to be able to move out of that chair." "We won't have to do anything for weeks!" My two boys were hoping for a break or that I'd be too out of it to notice them slacking off.

Meal Planning

Planning how you are going to feed yourself and your family takes some real thought. Of course you can eat Domino's delivery for six weeks, but even the most hard-core pizza lover is going to rebel. You can enlist your friends and family to deliver dinner each night, but that will take coordination and a spreadsheet program. It's nice to have your friends deliver a home-cooked meal once or twice a week -- there's nothing like homemade pork tenderloin, mashed potatoes and steamed asparagus when someone else prepares it for you. You can make meals ahead of your surgical date and freeze them. You can hire someone to do your grocery shopping and make sure your spouse or children know how to cook certain easy meals. You can use a service like GrubHub.com where you order take-out meals from participating restaurants in your town -- order your favorite restaurant meals and have them delivered right to your door. Or purchase a whole bunch of pre-fab meals and store them in your freezer.

Subscription Meal Services, Online Grocery Shopping and Meal Delivery

If you have a family member who likes to cook, there are online subscription meal services like Blue Apron, Plated, HelloFresh, Home Chef and PeachDish. Professional chefs design healthy and delicious recipes, shop for everything you need to make the meal, complete with seasonings, and the fresh ingredients are delivered to your door. These ingredients are shipped in a way which will keep them fresh for 24 hours in case you aren't home when they are delivered, and last up to four to five days in the refrigerator. It costs about $9-$10 per person.

Another option is Schwan's online grocery shopping and home delivery service. You can choose from more than 350 family favorites which are flash frozen for freshness and flavor, including breakfast, lunch, dinner and snack foods. Place your order online or via your phone and choose your delivery date. Lots of choices, very affordable and you never left your recliner!

The online grocery shopping and subscription food services are a big help to your spouse because he or she doesn't have to shop for all the ingredients. Everything needed for the meal arrives ready for the chef to begin cooking. If you feel like it, walk into the kitchen and enjoy just watching the process. You don't want to even think about engaging that shoulder until you have been advised that it's okay by your doctor. Bon Apetit!

Prime Pantry by Amazon Prime

For your dry goods, canned goods, cleaning supplies and paper products, Amazon Prime has designed a way to make your recovery even more enjoyable. Prime Pantry offers hundreds of brand-name everyday items in normal sizes at reasonable prices. They do the heavy lifting and ship it all to you for $5.99 per Prime Pantry box. You can order what you need, when you need. You are not going to be able to go out and shop for a long time. This is a great option that allows you to do your grocery shopping in your pajamas with your shoulder safely snuggled in pillows. Place items in your online digital cart and watch your Prime Pantry box fill up on your computer screen. Amazon will tell you what percentage of the box you have filled. Purchase as much or as little as you need. You will need an Amazon Prime Membership to take advantage of Prime Pantry.

Paper Products, Dirty Dishes and Crock Pots

Have plenty of paper plates, bowls and cups so dishes don't get backed up. Dirty dishes are annoying when you can't do anything about them. Let them be dirty in the dishwasher, not on the counter where you have to see them. Keep pressing "Rinse Hold" until you have enough to run a load. Keep the paper products on the counter in reach. It's easier to fix yourself a snack when everything you need is in plain sight and you don't have to worry about washing up. Time enough for that when you have two working arms again.

Meals were a concern for me. I like to cook. I like sitting down to home-cooked meals. I was overwhelmed at the thought of pre-making food. I like to shop the same day I cook, then invent and make it up as I go. I don't follow recipes. I had to kick perfectionism to the curb in this area because Seal-A-Meal and I are not friends. There was nothing more unappetizing to me than a frozen block of greyish food. Crock pots and I are sworn enemies. I have purchased over 10 crock pots in my life. After making nasty messes each time, I gave them away.

I tried. I really tried. Sort of. I made and froze a week's worth of dinners to get started. I froze mashed potatoes (don't freeze mashed potatoes...ever!...when they thaw, they resemble white vomit), Chicken and Vegetable casserole, Spaghetti and Meat Sauce, Chicken A La King, Beef Stew and Vegetable Soup. Too much work for so little output. There was way too much Pyrex in the freezer. I pre-purchased lots of frozen ready-made meals, extra snacks and extra household supplies. I bought so much stuff -- Hungry Man dinners, Stouffer's Lasagnas, frozen pizzas -- because I was nervous about the surgery. I figured if I died, at least they would eat.

Household Chores

Have some practice days where you pretend your arm is immobilized to see where the holes are in your family's daily habits. That's always eye-opening. See what needs to be taught and/or tightened up regarding chores. You can even purchase a sling and an immobilizer to wear. This is crazy, stressful and not fun at all. "Mom's cheating!" I am not!" "Honey, this is not a game!" "Actually it is, I haven't had the surgery yet!!!" Still getting your family to play along can be helpful -- part of them will be nervous about you being out of commission and the other part will be silently celebrating their anticipated freedom.

Replace sheets and blankets with easy-to-pull-up comforters and duvet covers to streamline bed making. Have everyone learn the laundry routine from hamper to drawer --- folding optional! Have your family practice loading and unloading the dishwasher. If you have a weekend helper, teach them exactly how to strip the beds and remake them, clean the bathrooms and kitchen, and vacuum -- all to your specifications. This may sound extreme, but it goes a long way in helping calm your nerves before surgery.

Schedules, organization, routines and systems will make the first bumpy days of your recovery that much smoother. This will be a big surrender on your part as you wrestle daily with frustration and dependence. Each day will bring new ways to come to terms with your limitations and get used to asking for help...from fixing meals to washing your hair to changing the toilet paper roll.

Subscriptions and Services

There are many subscriptions and services available which will make your recovery at home more enjoyable. Amazon Prime costs $99 per year and gives you free second day shipping on most items, lots of great movies and tv shows to watch on Amazon Instant Video and you can borrow books from the Kindle Owner's lending library. Netflix costs $7.99 a month and offers DVD rentals and streaming video-on-demand service. You can watch tv shows, movies and lots of good documentaries. Gaiam TV costs $9.95 per month and offers unlimited access to inspirational films, yoga and fitness videos, and original shows on various spiritual, esoteric and just plain "out there" topics. Some of their shows and documentaries have merit and some are a little freaky. You have to decide for yourself but it sure is entertaining while you are deciding. You might decide "no, I don't think that I am a descendent of an alien" but you might say "hey, sticking my feet in the dirt might be a viable way to heal my plantar fasciitis with the healing energy of the planet." Stranger things have happened. If you have a ROKU, you can subscribe to all of these and many more.

What the Heck are You Gonna Wear?

Finding sling-friendly clothing that doesn't rub against your incision, isn't too tight and isn't irritating to wear all day and all night is an adventure with shoulder surgery. Purchase everything oversized and loose so it will go on easily. If you are female, you probably aren't going to want to wear bra straps for a while because of your incision. Some folks wear oversize button-up shirts because you can hang your arm down and not disturb your shoulder while putting it on. Short-sleeved ones are a better option because you aren't dealing with all that extra sleeve that has to be buttoned or rolled up. But buttons are an issue...you will need someone to help you in and out of the shirt. You just want to be comfortable. Dressing in all cotton is helpful because it breathes better. Sweatpants or pajama pants? Socks or no socks? Bra or no bra? There are many options. Decide what will work best for you.

Ready-Made Shirts

ShoulderShirts on Etsy has t-shirts that open up at both shoulders with velcro. DressWithEase on Etsy has shirts that are cut up the side and under the sleeve on the side where your sling is. You can purchase them with little Velcro tabs or you could sew little Velcro tabs on yourself. The shirts at DressWithEase are custom made when you order them. All these shirts can run from $30 - $50. On Amazon, there are men's and women's easy on and off shoulder surgery t-shirts by a company called BlossomBreeze. These t-shirts also have velcro seals at the shoulders and upper arms, are 100% cotton and are nice-looking. They run about $35 each.

Make Your Own Shirts

Velcro is frustrating to line up correctly and stick together when you're dealing with only one arm. It can also feel like too much pressure on your incision site in the first few weeks. Yes, you want to look nice and put together, but face it, you just had shoulder surgery. You don't want to move your arm at all in the beginning. One way around this is to purchase some oversize t-shirts from Walmart or Target. Figure out which side your sling will be on. Cut the t-shirt on the seam from the bottom of the shirt all the way up the side under the armpit to the end of the sleeve. Stick your good arm through the full sleeve, drag the neck opening over your head with your good arm and let the other side drape over your shoulder and sling like a poncho. No pressure, no irritation plus you are warm and covered. The t-shirts cost about $5-$6 apiece and you don't feel bad using scissors on them. Also, they are soft and not constricting in any way.

Button-Up Shirts

Sometime during your first six weeks you will be ready for the button-up shirt. A men's large short-sleeved button-up shirt works well once you are comfortable and have mastered the art of taking your sling on and off. Always start with your repair arm first. With your repair arm hanging down at your side, draw the sleeve up and over your hand, all the way up your arm until it is up on your shoulder. Once that sleeve is up on the repair arm, you can bend your good arm and stick it through the other sleeve. You may need help buttoning for several weeks. Loose-fitting all-cotton shirts are much more comfortable than a trim, form-fitting cotton/spandex blouse. There's plenty of time for cute fashion in the future. Right now you don't want anything that will rub on your incision or make you sweat uncomfortably in your sling.

A Real T-Shirt with Sides

It's a big day when you slip on a real t-shirt for the first time since the surgery. Go for an oversize one so you don't get all tangled up getting in. Begin with your repair arm. Keeping your repair arm down at your side, gently slip the armhole of the t-shirt over your hand and slide it all the way up. Next, slip your head into the neck hole and settle the arm and shoulder section of the t-shirt into place over your repair. Finally, take your good arm and put it through the other armhole. You are dressed in your first t-shirt of your recovery! I was conservative and went slowly in my clothing journey. I didn't want to get my arm caught in a bad position. The homemade t-shirt poncho can actually be usable after you are out of the sling by simply tying the two cut ends of the shirt together in a knot on the side, Daisy Duke style. It's a way to get a little more life out of the t-shirts and wear them without exposing your whole side.

The Bra

For the first few weeks of recovery you can purchase a camisole bra with spaghetti straps that you can step into, haul up your body and over your breasts to cover yourself. No matter what your size, it isn't about support in the beginning – just comfort and coverage. Put the strap on your good shoulder and pull up the other side to just under your armpit, covering your boob, and leave the unused strap hanging or snip it off altogether.

After the first few weeks, it is all about THE BRA or lack of one. If you are like me and have a bust size that is 36D or larger, THE BRA is going to dominate your thinking. Dressing the ladies is going to be an ongoing challenge. From all-cotton t-shirt camisoles with one strap cut off to an all-cotton strapless that has to be modified to stay up and not roll into a squeegee underneath your breast to a steel-belted radial strapless to hold you up and in place for that first social outing – it's an experience.

My one-strap camisole bra struggled when it came to coverage during physical therapy. I purchased some all-cotton strapless bras. When they wouldn't stay in place, I came up with the bright idea of safety-pinning the strapless bra to my shirt -- sort of an all-in-one bra-shirt thing to keep everything stationery. Unfortunately, the weight of my boobs pulled on the neck of my button-up shirt making me all constricted and unable to move easily in any direction. My physical therapist remarked that I seemed tense and uncomfortable with my routine that day. I was too mortified to tell her I was being held captive by my own medieval torture shirt. I fixed the problem by cinching in the sides of the strapless bra with safety pins to make it snug and roll-proof by the next PT session. I confessed the bra fiasco when she noticed I was doing better and seemed much more relaxed. She just laughed at me.

It's hard to find a comfortable, attractive bra with straps that doesn't give you a horrible headache by late afternoon. Shoulder surgery makes straps painfully impossible for at least the first four months. I didn't wear my first bra with straps until five months out. I did a ton of research to find a bra that put the least amount of stress on my shoulder. A front-closure, support bra with straps that could detach in front was the first bra I could wear without pain for long periods of time. One style was workable, came in pretty colors and floral patterns and had a nice lift and separate effect as opposed to a squashed monoboob. Another style wasn't my cup of tea, but would work in a pinch. It didn't have detachable, adjustable shoulder straps. Also, it created a pointy 1950's look – add some pedal pushers and you're good to go!

I ordered my favorite bra from Amazon. I decided the only way I could take pressure off my shoulder was with a posture support bra. It's called the Comfort Choice Bra. It comes in a variety of colors. It's a wireless front-hook closure posture support bra with cushioned adjustable front hook straps. Those front hook straps are a lifesaver when your shoulder starts to ache or you are having ultrasound done on your shoulder and you don't feel like taking off your whole bra. The strap unhooks very quickly and easily. If you are driving in the car and your shoulder feels uncomfortable, you can unhook it, release the pressure and nothing moves or slips around on you. Great bra!

The Glamorise Magic Lift wireless front hook posture bra was the 1950's throwback a la Peggy Sue Got Married and didn't have the neato front hook bra straps. It was comfortable, though. It's a good back-up bra. You can purchase this bra on Amazon as well. Each bra runs about $30 - $35.

If you need a good strapless bra to wear to a function or event before you can even contemplate the thought of any strap on your shoulder or resting on your incision cite, Wacoal makes an amazing one. The Wacoal Women's Plus-Size Full Figure Red Carpet Strapless Bra is available on Amazon for $60.00. It magically stays up with an iron grip that makes you feel completely secure and gives you a nice shape.

My friend's wedding was the day right after the six-week mark: May 23, 2015. I had big plans. I wanted a new dress and a real bra that lifted and separated, not just a smoosh and push. Since I could only hang my arm down to get dressed and a button-up shirt was the most comfortable, I needed a shirt dress. No belt, no complications -- just an oversize shirt that went all the way to the floor and looked lovely. Not too much to ask! I found one that would work. It was lightweight, all cotton and didn't hurt to put on. Problem solved, I moved on to THE BRA. I found the strapless feat of engineering made by Wacoal that was pricey, but looked like it would do the trick. Fingers crossed, I ordered it.

THE BRA arrived the day before the wedding. I prayed it would work. I enlisted my hapless husband to put me into this strapless wonder. Working together and trying not to disturb my repair, we filled the cups and raised them skyward. Now for the hooks. He carefully tried to make the two sides come together in the back and latch. He was scared he was going to hurt me and I was just as scared he wasn't going to be able to hook the damn bra. Then I'd never make it to the wedding because my new giant purple dress wouldn't work without a firm foundation! Once in, I was feeling good. I hadn't seen my boobs that happy in weeks. I felt like a million bucks! In fact I had such a good time being out with people and eating different foods that I didn't go home until the clean-up crew physically took the table down in front of me and asked me for my chair.

Daily Apres Surgery Ready-To-Wear

Plan your daily after surgery wardrobe. Include underpants, socks, pajama pants/yoga pants/sweats (with easy-to-pull-up elastic waists), modified camisole bras, and modified t-shirts or button-up shirts. Pull them all out (at least seven days worth) and pile them in a waist-high area in a corner of your bedroom in full view for easy access. Keep them there for the duration. A good place to put them is on top of a desk or dresser. Separate them into piles by category for easy selection. When ready, choose an outfit from the different piles and place the pieces on the bed for the actual moment of dressing. Everything needs to be within easy reach – drawers are hard/impossible to pull and you will feel the stress all the way over on your surgery side. Closets are hard to navigate with a sling. I have a narrow "chuck and stuff" closet that takes two good arms to find anything. My idea of putting clothes on the top shelf is to take aim, fire toward the center and hope something sticks -- not good with a sling. Closets and dresser drawers are not surgery friendly. You might as well lock up all your clothes and throw away the key for all the good it will do you -- your bedroom has to be user-friendly.

Shoes

You can use SOFSOLE Performance Lace stretch laces on your sneakers or HICKIES which is a no-tie shoelace replacement that turns any sneaker into a slip-on. Now you don't have to worry about tying them or asking anyone else to tie them for you. Lots of people wear orthotics or just feel more secure in their sneakers. It's very important that you wear shoes that are supportive and keep you securely on your feet when you walk. You must not fall. Falling is dangerous. It's the quickest way to undo your repair. Do everything in your power to stay on your feet.

Your Recovery Nest

Whether it's your spouse, a friend or a hired caregiver, make sure someone will drive you to the hospital the morning of the surgery. This caregiver should stay during the surgery, get all instructions for after surgery care and follow-up appointments, bring you back home from surgery and settle you back down in your house or apartment. You'll feel like a petted poodle coming home from the vet's, but it will help your anxicty to havo someone take care of all the details. You won't be in any shape to do this for yourself.

It's important to map out your house, especially any stairs. Staying on all one level is much easier if you can manage it. If your bedroom is upstairs, think about setting it up downstairs. During the first six weeks, if you have to navigate any stairs in order to get to your doctor appointments or to physical therapy, you need to be heavily supervised. Guard against falling at all costs because that can undo your repair in an instant and you'll be back at square one. And that means saying "No, I can't do that." Or "No, I can't be there at this time." Or "Thank you for the invitation to lunch. I'm going to have to take a rain check until after my six-week visit with the surgeon." Saying no is hard because you don't want to be a baby or a spoilsport and not check out the new Italian restaurant with your friends. Guess what? You just had shoulder surgery – you get to be a baby, if only for a little bit! Let them bring you take-out and tell you all about it. This is your time to heal and protect that repair.

Last Minute Preparations

You may wake up from surgery and find yourself in a

shoulder cryo cuff which is a motorized cooler that pumps fresh ice water every 20 minutes thru tubes to ice packs on your shoulder that never need to be moved. If not, and you are interested in one, you can order one from Amazon or Ebay. Talk to your doctor and see if you need one. Make sure you test it and it works properly before you need to use it. Otherwise, regular ice packs work well. Have several in the freezer ready to go. You'll want to be able to switch them out at regular intervals.

Are you anxious about being in a recliner chair all night on medication while everyone in the house is sleeping? What if you have to go to the bathroom but you can't or are afraid to get out of the recliner and you have an accident? No one likes to think about it but it can happen. Not only would you be a mess and have to change when you are wet and sleepy, but someone would have to clean the chair so you could rest again. Just get a package of Depends and wear one for the first few days. If you don't need it, don't use it! At least it's there for that hypothetical "what if?"

Arrange your living area exactly as you need it to be since you will be inhabiting it for a few weeks. Set up a basket to hold your eyeglasses, remotes, a book or Kindle, tissues and anything else you need within reach.

Make sure you have lots of extra pillows and blankets. Put a large bag of Lifesavers in your basket to suck on because being intubated can leave you with a sore throat. You shouldn't take pain medication on an empty stomach. Put some granola bars or pre-packaged snacks in your basket, too. Can you see the television from your recliner? Is your recliner out of the high traffic part of the room? You want to be safe and tucked in so no one can bump your chair.

Vitamins, Supplements and OTC Medications

Lots of vitamins and supplements can help you heal. These include Vitamin E with tocopherols, Vitamin C, Vitamin D, Vitamin B, zinc, magnesium and more. While it's optimum to get these vitamins and minerals from your food, it's harder after surgery when you can't cook or shop for yourself. There is lots of good information to read and study about what is best for your body after surgery.

High Gamma Vitamin E with mixed tocopherols is an antioxidant that protects cell membranes and other fat-soluble parts of the body. It can help reduce scar tissue, reduces inflammation and helps to prevent adhesions forming after surgery. Check with your doctor if this form of Vitamin E is right for you. Vitamin C is an antioxidant that helps boost your body's immune system, promotes healing and helps make collagen. Vitamin D is good for bone healing and muscle function. Vitamin B helps reduce inflammation and promote healing. Zinc helps speed healing, reduces inflammation and helps reduce scar tissue formation. Magnesium helps your body deal with the stress that surgery can cause.

Getting enough protein in your diet after shoulder surgery is important. Tendons are formed from collagen. Protein fibers form collagen and collagen forms together to make the connective tissue in muscles and tendons that hold us together. After your shoulder repair, you want to do all you can to help the tendon grow to the bone with proper tensile strength. Also, protein will help the surrounding muscles get strong and healthy as you work in physical therapy. Protein powder is a good supplement in addition to other protein in your diet. You can mix it into yogurt or a smoothie to make it more palatable.

The first few days after surgery you'll be on heavy pain medications. Your doctor wants you to be comfortable and fairly sedated so you don't move that shoulder. It needs rest and quiet. Pain medications often have the unwelcome side effect of constipation. This happens because not only are you sedated and slowed down, but so is your colon. Everything slows down. Your doctor may recommend you begin taking a product like MiraLAX a few days before your surgery to make sure you are regular. MiraLAX is a gentle stool softener that's used to relieve occasional constipation and irregularity. It dissolves completely in any beverage and is sugar-free. If that doesn't work and you are having difficulty having a bowel movement, Dulcolax is recommended. It's also a stool softener, but much more of a heavy gun. You don't want to be constipated with a shoulder repair; straining to go puts a strain on the shoulder. You need everything moving smoothly, especially your bowels! If you don't need it and you are the whiz king or queen, more power to you -- but if not, you'll regret not having it on hand.

Arnica is a homeopathic medication made from the alpine plant Arnica Montana or Mountain Daisy. It has noticeable healing properties and is recommended by many professionals, including homeopaths and acupuncturists, for post-surgical swelling and bruising to help shorten recovery time. It's worth reading about and seeing if it has any merit for you. You can get it at your local health food store.

Ibuprofen or other anti-inflammatory medications like

naproxen aren't recommended for the first six to twelve weeks because they can interfere with your tendon growth. Your doctor will go over this with you. Your surgeon will prescribe pain medications. Tylenol is okay to take because it's not an anti-inflammatory.

Chapter 3:

PRACTICE, PRACTICE, PRACTICE!

Dominant Arm or Non-Dominant Arm

Recovery from shoulder surgery is time-consuming and difficult. If your surgery is on your non-dominant arm, it'll be easier. Fifteen years ago I broke my dominant arm. I had a cast on for six months after surgery to install a metal plate. It was hard to carry out daily tasks with my non-dominant arm. I learned how to diaper my baby with my non-dominant hand and my teeth. Writing, eating, brushing my teeth, getting dressed and wiping my rear end was a real pain. However by the end of the six months, I was a pro -- due to practice!

It's not easy to ask for help all the time. You don't want to be beholden to anyone or be a burden in any way. Shoulder surgery changes all of that in an instant. You are weak, completely dependent in many ways and you need all the helping hands you can get! This is why practice prior to the surgery is so important. Practice helps you regain some independence.

If the surgery will be on your dominant arm, practice with your non-dominant hand for as long as you can before surgery. Pain coupled with an inability to crumple toilet paper into an adequate mass in order to sufficiently clean your bottom is an unwelcome experience. Even though my surgery was going to be on my non-dominant side, I followed the advice of my sister and practiced with one hand doing all these things until I was a pro.

Toothpaste and Floss

Putting toothpaste on your toothbrush with only one hand is hard. Putting the tube of toothpaste between your knees and twisting off the cap without squirting toothpaste across the room is an art. Holding the tube of toothpaste with one hand and using your teeth to unscrew the cap is another talent you can develop! You can't floss with regular floss. Buy floss sticks. Practice opening the bag to get one out. Soon you'll say "the hell with this!" and just throw them loose in a drawer. All these details seem laughable until you can't get your floss stick out of the little ziplock baggy. They all fall out on the floor where the dog had a pee accident and you burst into tears because your arm hurts and you can't manage the tiniest detail.

You and Your Toilet

When you sit down on the toilet, on which side is the toilet paper? Reaching across your body to grab the toilet paper can cause pain. Make sure the toilet paper dispenser is on the correct side you need. If it isn't, get a stand-alone toilet paper holder that you can move anywhere you want. Have you thought about toilet seat height? I got a raised toilet seat because my sister reminded me you don't realize how far down you have to go to sit and do your business until you're in pain in a sling with stitches. The extra four inches you don't have to travel downward is heaven sent. I purchased the simple raised toilet seat from Walmart. It costs around $25-$30. In order to install the raised toilet seat, you have to put up your regular toilet seat. That becomes what you lean against. If it is stained, old and unsightly, replace your regular toilet seat with a fresh one so you are not leaning against ickiness. Small details like this mean a lot when you are feeling vulnerable. And vulnerable gets a whole new meaning after surgery.

Using a flushable cleansing wipe is beyond helpful when you're weak as a kitten, but you have to use the litter box. However, be forewarned that constant use of these wipes can irritate, causing itching and burning which is fresh hell when you are in a sling. If you have a bidet, use it! If you don't have that option, use Aleva Bamboo baby wipes with calendula to help soothe those angry tissues. These are available on Amazon for $30 for six packages of eighty wipes each.

Take Your Time -- Modify, Modify, Modify!

You are used to being in charge of your life and going where you want, when you want. You will still be able to do that but with modifications. The biggest modification is giving yourself enough time. No matter how much you have practiced your daily habits of going to the bathroom, brushing your teeth, brushing your hair or changing your clothes, it is completely a new set of rules when you come home from surgery and you are in your big pillow support sling and attached to your cryo cuff. Surgery is flat-out exhausting. Going to the bathroom involves getting up, shuffling down the hall to the bathroom with someone helping you by holding your good arm, pulling your pants down, bending your knees and making it to a sitting down position. And that doesn't include wiping, flushing and getting those pants back up in order to make it back down the hall to your recliner chair. It is all doable, but you must give yourself enough time and not be angry that it isn't all just a breeze. It's not. Your shoulder is the joint with the most amount of motion that allows you to do just about anything. When it is out of commission, your world gets real small, real fast. That's okay. This learning curve is only for six weeks. During those six weeks you will make modest strides each day, getting more confident and competent.

Getting Dressed

After the surgery, allow yourself enough time to get dressed. You no longer have the option of hopping on one foot while you try to shove the other one through the leg hole of your underpants. Every piece of clothing from the skin out requires your full concentration and attention to detail so you don't move your arm the wrong way or lose your balance. It's all fun and games until you can't pull your sweatpants out from the bottom of the stack of unorganized clothes with your one good hand without dumping them all on the floor. You'll just leave them because you're too damn tired to pick them up again.

When you are ready to dress, put your freshly picked

clothes on the bed and SIT DOWN next to them. Lay a
towel down on the bed if a naked bottom gives you the
squirmies. Put one foot through the underpants leg hole,
then the other one. When you have pulled them up to
knee height, you may stand up to pull them up the rest of
the way as long as you are right next to the bed. If you
get a toe stuck or start to sway, you can sit right back
down on the bed again. Do the same routine with your
pants. Get them on as far as you can sitting down, then
stand up to pull them up the rest of the way. Be ready to
sit down if you lose your balance. Make sure to rest
between articles of clothing. This isn't a contest. No one
is keeping track of how fast you can dress. No one cares.
All anyone cares about is that you don't stress out and
jeopardize your repair.

One Hand Products

There are many new products out on the market that
are helpful when you only have one good hand to use.
WrightStuff.biz has lots of adaptive kitchen aids you can
look into purchasing. Rocker knives give you the ability to
cut your own food with one hand. There are jar openers,
bag openers and bottle openers. You can stick the jar or
bottle between your knees and try to open it with one
hand, but you run the risk of dousing yourself with pickle

juice or wearing the salad dressing. Better to invest in a few non-slip, grippy openers than having to keep changing your clothes. There are also non-slip mats that help keep your food from sliding off your tray and into your lap. There is even an electric can opener designed to open cans with one hand.

Fiskar scissors cut well with either hand. You can find coffee cups that have a handle on both sides. There are leather weights to put down on your bills to keep them in place or keep a file open while you are working. Cool sponges on a stick hold a bar of soap so you can soap up your own back in the shower with one hand while sitting on your bath chair. A bath chair is a necessity for your first showers. You can sit safely and rest your repair arm in your lap during your shower.

When it comes to personal hygiene in the bathroom, there is a handy dandy bottom wiper stick called the Self Wipe Toilet Aid with a button you press that releases the soiled toilet paper into the toilet bowl. You can find this at RehabMart.com. If you are one of the lucky ones whose surgery is done on your non-dominant side, you can't imagine purchasing this. But if you have surgery on your dominant side, you are probably going "hmmmmm." It's all out there -- whatever you need to accomplish your daily personal hygiene. I won't lie to you. It all costs money. However all these items are health care items for use during your recovery from surgery. They can be deducted as medical expenses on your income taxes.

How Am I Gonna Bathe and Shower?

If you are female, consider a really short haircut. Not only is brushing your hair difficult, but after you have shoulder surgery? Hair washing, showering and bathing is akin to rocket science. You can ask someone to help wash your hair, but it gets really dicey because there's no getting around that shoulder. You don't want anyone except your doctor or physical therapist anywhere near your shoulder. With super short hair you can easily "wash" it with a baby wipe or damp washcloth using only one hand.

I have chia head hair that is thick and grows fast. I'm not really attached to my hair so I wanted to cut it all off or go bald and draw designs on my head. My husband said "no bald head." I told my hairdresser to cut my hair really short. A sharp, pointy, "hair as weapon" look. I wanted to look fierce and scrappy. I wanted courage.

Baby wipes are great for freshening up armpits and

crotches. There are cleansing washcloths and dry shampoos. Make sure you have lots of clean outfits and underwear. You can put off the big shower day for a week or so...until you are very steady on your feet and can take your sling on and off with confidence. It's not a race. It's not a beauty contest. Your repair is held in place by anchors and sutures. Your reattachment depends on your making sure no harm comes to the repair. Anything that involves water and slippery surfaces can lead to a fall. Your shoulder does not care if your hair is greasy or if your legs look as if you are wearing hairy knee socks. Its tensile strength needs six whole weeks of babying to mature through Phase One. Don't screw it up for the sake of vanity.

In order to feel clean and fresh before your first shower, you can purchase Comfort Bath Personal Cleansing Ultra-Thick Disposable Washcloths. You can get four packs of eight washcloths for about $16. These disposable washcloths can be warmed in the microwave. It's simple to thoroughly sponge bathe all the body parts you can reach with one hand (because you practiced, remember?). You can also purchase a large supply of baby wipes to clean your face, neck, armpits, bottom, crotch, legs and feet in a pinch if you just want to feel fresh but aren't up to microwaving your disposable bath washcloths just yet. Be cautious with bathing. Better to be dirty and grow plants all over your body like bad Mrs. Piggle-Wiggle children than risk a fall.

Showering

Eventually you will need a real shower. After wiping down your hair with baby wipes for the first few days and washing your hair with one hand and a washcloth in the kitchen sink for another week, you'll be more than ready. You'll be sticky and itchy with perfumy sweat. Your first shower will be a challenge. It's a good idea to have many rehearsals while fully dressed. Plan to have someone present on emergency duty to rescue you if you get into trouble. If you're showering in the first couple of days, make sure you cover your incision area with a waterproof band aid or plastic wrap to keep it dry. After your first doctor's appointment, they will let you know when you can shower without protecting the incision.

I was panicky about my first shower. Your physical therapist will help you realize you can take a shower by showing you how to take off the sling. She will talk your inner jumper down and explain how to place your arm in the shower, either resting in your lap or hanging gently down at your side. Learning how to take off my sling and beginning my range of motion exercises were the first steps toward unlocking my anxiety cage.

My first physical therapy session was on Day 18 after my surgery. I waited almost three weeks to take a real shower. I needed to be clean. I couldn't face them without a shower. I wasn't a brave person at all. A brave person would go in with greasy warrior chicken hair, braided armpits and smelling like last week's lunch. I didn't want to be that person in physical therapy with the bad smell that people smile kindly at but won't sit next to.

Since my fall in the shower, I am skittish around showers and bathtubs. We have a 1930's house. It has a big, deep bathtub with a shower nozzle. I've used a shower chair since I fell. You can purchase a shower chair or bench with a back from Amazon, Walmart or your local drugstore for about $35-$40. The one I use doesn't have arms. The arms would be too difficult to maneuver around in a sling. If you have a walk-in shower, then place the shower chair in it and step in carefully. The following steps are if you live in a house or apartment with only a tub shower.

TIME TO SHOWER (using a tub)

Do the following 7 steps **WITHOUT WATER**:

Step 1: Get someone to put the shower chair into the shower facing the shower nozzle.

Step 2: Get same someone to put another sturdy chair of the same height on the outside of the tub facing the same way as the shower chair.

Step 3: While fully dressed and still in your sling, sit on chair outside the tub. Rest.

Step 4: Practice swinging leg closest to tub over the side of the tub in front of shower chair.

Step 5: Using good arm to steady yourself, maneuver your bottom from outside chair to inside chair slowly, one cheek at a time. When both bottom cheeks are on the shower chair, gently pull outer leg over the side of the tub into shower. Rest.

Step 6: Reverse the process.

Step 7: Repeat as often as necessary until you're confident you can do it naked with a vulnerable arm.

Time to ADD WATER:

Step 8: While fully dressed in your sling and standing on the outside of the tub in your non-skid shoes, practice turning on the shower to the desired water temperature. Turn it off.

Step 9: Hang your towel on the back of the outside

chair. Leave the bathroom and head for the bedroom.

Step 10: Take off t-shirt poncho and pajama pants with good hand, shimmy out of underwear. Take off shoes and socks. Put on non-skid shower shoes.

Step 11: Sit naked on bed. By this time you know all the ins and outs of your sling. Sit on the bed, unbuckle the shoulder strap, unbuckle the waist strap and let the whole contraption slip off you onto the bed without moving your body. Pretty damn tricky.

Step 12: Leaving sling on the bed, carefully walk to chair on the outside of the tub, turn on water to desired temp. My shower is such that I can turn it off and turn it on again in about a minute and the water temp is still the same. I turned the water off, and sat down in the outside chair with my arm in "invisible sling position", close to my body. I didn't want to fuss with a separate sling for the shower because I had no desire to learn another sling and I couldn't get my fancy one wet.

Using steps 1-7, get yourself seated on the shower chair in the tub and turn on the pre-warmed shower water with your good hand. Be careful when you soap your rear end -- you don't want to slide off your shower chair!

Your first shower will be unbelievably sweet. Sit there

and let warm water cascade over you while you bliss out in a major way. Dump a little shampoo on your head with one hand and wash your hair. If your shampoo bottle has a cap, hold the bottle between your knees while you twist the cap off with your non-repair hand. Tip the bottle to get a little shampoo out, then rub it on your head. Put the cap back on while the bottle is still between your knees. A squirt bottle might be easier. Make sure you have the shampoo all ready to go before you get in the shower. To wash the armpit under your operated shoulder, bend over at the waist and let the arm passively come away from your body and hang down. You can safely wash under your arm in this position. It's the same position as the pendulum exercises your physical therapist will have you do.

Make sure you have someone within hollering distance. Have them check on you several times. After you turn off the water, reach for your towel from the back of the outside chair with your good arm. Gently pat yourself dry as much as you can while sitting on the bath chair. When you are ready, hang the towel on the back of the outside chair and slowly reverse the getting in process. Soon you'll be sitting on the outside chair. Carefully make your way back to the bedroom and put on your sling. It will feel so good to put it back on, knowing your shoulder is back in its protective cocoon.

First Bath

Taking your first bath is completely different than taking your first shower. With a bath chair, an extra chair on the outside of the tub and a well-practiced routine, a shower can be handled more easily than a tub bath. I didn't attempt a tub bath until halfway through Phase Two, six to twelve weeks after surgery. Use a chair on the outside of the tub for balance and hang onto it with your good arm. Practice getting in a dry tub with your clothes and sling on. You can take off your shoes or not. You will feel like an idiot but do it anyway. Position yourself in the tub. Figure out the best way to place your arm to keep your shoulder protected. Doing this for the first time while naked is not a good idea. Again, make sure someone is nearby while you are taking a bath for the first time after surgery. They'll need to check on you and, if necessary, help heave you out again. Kiss your modesty goodbye, folks...after shoulder surgery, nothing's sacred.

Have your towel ready where you can reach it next to the bathtub. When you feel confident, strip off your clothes and your sling (you won't have to worry about that if you wait as long as I did!). Step into a dry tub. No water until you're safely sitting down. Lower yourself to your knees, carefully lean with your good arm against the side of the tub and somehow skootch your bottom to the side and unfold your legs. Add water once you're settled.

When you are done, empty all the water out of the tub while you are still sitting down. Carefully reverse the skootching and leaning with your good arm until you are back on your knees. For the first few times, until you are confident, have someone assist you out of the tub. When you think you can handle it on your own, be mindful and watch your footing. If you need a support or chair on the outside of the tub to help you get out, position it where you need it before you get in.

When I got in the tub the first time, I ended up facing the wrong way. Don't know how it happened. Turning around was like trying to back a horse up into a mini-van. But I was determined. My first bath felt as though someone had poured champagne all over my skin. I didn't want to get out. Truth was, I didn't know how to get out. Which is why I say practice. Because I didn't. I was stuck in the tub and I had to yell for help. Not my finest moment.

Where Am I Going to Sleep?

Figure out where you are going to sleep. Every blog post and message concerning shoulder surgery discussed how painful and uncomfortable it was to sleep after the surgery. The consensus: a recliner was the best way to go.

Most people who have shoulder surgery will sleep in the recliner chair afterward, some as long as five to six weeks. There are so many options out there: leather, upholstered, levers on either side, remote controls to open and close the chair, big ones, little ones, all-in-one-footrests and every price imaginable. If you don't have one and don't want to spend the money on one, you can borrow one. Rearrange your living space to accommodate the chair for your optimum comfort. You're going to be in it for a while; you may as well be happy. If you live alone, please consider one with a remote control so you can get in and out of it without trouble. If you get one with a lever, make sure it is not on the same side as your repair. That's a disaster waiting to happen! You'll be stuck in the chair if you don't have someone to help you in or out because you can't use your repair side at all and you won't be able to expend the energy to push it closed with your legs. Also, using your legs could possibly pull on your repair.

Even if a recliner chair looks really comfy, it's not comfy after two hours and can get down right painful after a night of sleeping in one. You'll need lots of pillows to cushion all the different parts of you and to cushion/support your arm. You'll also want to support your lower back and your neck because all sorts of chiropractic issues can arise due to bad sleeping positions. You don't need any unnecessary pain.

I purchased a Sunshine Pillow Chiropractic Neck Support Pillow and a Homedics OT-LUM Therapy Lumbar Cushion Support Pillow with a velour cover, both from Amazon. I also placed a Coccyx Gel Seat Cushion with Fleece Top, also from Amazon, in the seat of the recliner. Practice sitting with your pillows and supports. Arrange them to your liking. Discard the ones that don't work and try something else. Also, try sleeping in the chair for a night so you can be sure you have all the pillows/supports you need.

If you live alone, please consider having a friend or relative stay with you for the first three to four days. You shouldn't be alone. There are too many things you will need assistance with and there's always the possibility of falling, especially during those first few days of round-the-clock pain medications. Having someone sleep in the same room with you is comforting and reassuring. You're vulnerable after surgery. Having a caregiver with you helps relieve stress.

I Hate the Recliner; I Want to Sleep in My Own Bed

If you're sick and tired of sleeping in your recliner chair, there are ways to sleep in your own bed with the comfort of a recliner. The Jobri Spine Reliever Bed Wedge and the Jobri Spine Reliever Leg Wedge are available on Amazon. You can also order a Natural White Noise Sound Machine, the Marpac DOHM-DS. It's highly recommended with great reviews on Amazon. It'll help you get a restful night's sleep. It'll also help your spouse sleep through the many times you get in and out of bed in order to use the restroom at night.

When the Jobri Wedges arrive, set them up on the side of the bed that's the same side as your repair. Your arm can be propped up on pillows on the far side of the bed. You may not want your repair shoulder in the middle of the bed where your spouse could roll into you. If you sleep alone, either side of the bed will work. The Bed Wedge has two positions: one has you sitting up tall and the other has you more reclined. The Leg Wedge goes under your knees. I took the butt cushion from the recliner chair in the living room and put it between the Bed Wedge and the Leg Wedge like a bridge. Otherwise, there can be too much pressure on your tailbone. You wouldn't think it would be that much of a big deal, but it can be. Go for maximum comfort. Put a soft pillow against the Bed Wedge and a big squishy pillow on the side to support your repair arm. Are you afraid of tripping or bumping into things in the dark in order to climb into position on the bed? Leave the bathroom light on all night or get a good, bright nightlight so you will have enough light to navigate.

It's exciting to sleep in your own bed again after being in a recliner. Make sure you have an ice pack for your arm. You can get them at a local drugstore or order them online. You can purchase Thera-Med reusable cold packs or Colpac cold therapy packs from Amazon. Using your good arm and your knees, climb into your bed and gingerly crash land onto the butt cushion with your rear end. Lean carefully against the Bed Wedge and soft pillow and swing your legs over the Leg Wedge. Then smoosh, wiggle, rock and roll until all parts are in the correct position and you are lying on your back in your bed recliner. It takes a little practice. An audience is not recommended.

Place your neck support pillow under your neck. If it's too firm, remove some of the interior support stuff so it's more squashy. Unbuckle just the neck strap of the sling and gently support your repair arm with the big squishy pillow. Finally, place your ice pack on and you're ready to rest in your own bed! Until you have to use the bathroom...and reverse the whole process! It'll take some trial and error to find the right positioning for a good night's sleep. At first I thought the Bed Wedge in the sitting up position would be the best, but I was wrong. It was uncomfortable and I sat like a sleepless owl perched in a tall tree for half the night before I switched to the more reclined position. But it's all progress toward your independence. I was happier sleeping with my husband and my dog in my big bed instead of being a prisoner in the living room recliner chair. Since you have to sleep in the sling for six weeks, do what you can to make it bearable.

Lying Down Flat In Your Bed

When you feel comfortable and your doctor says it's okay, lying down flat in your bed is like Christmas, the lottery and sex all rolled up into one. People who can lie flat on their back without fear or pain totally take it for granted. You will need your giant squishy pillow to floonch up under your arm to support it in a comfortable position. Then pay the Sandman and head straight for Dreamland. And the day you can put on a real nightgown, real pajamas or sleep completely butt naked without that sling is another I kissed the cute boy on top of the Ferris Wheel day! All these milestones are reason enough to keep a big box of cupcakes in the fridge and have daily celebrations -- they are that big in your tiny little world of recovery.

Chapter 4:

SURGERY

The Night Before Surgery and You Have to Pack

Pack your bag with everything you will need after surgery. This includes your cool poncho T-shirt, cotton pajama bottoms or sweat pants, camisole bra with one strap cut off, fresh underwear or a Depends (or both!) and socks. Don't forget easy, slip-on shoes or your sneakers with the stretchy laces. Your surgeon will have thorough instructions for you regarding eating, drinking and your medications. Usually you will be told to stop eating and drinking by midnight or earlier, depending on how early your surgery is in the morning. Take a luxurious bath with bubbles or a really long hot shower. Get a good night's sleep in a comfy position. It will be a while for both!

I was hitting new levels of crazy with each tick of the

clock hand, talking myself down from canceling at the final hour. I had to go through with it now – I had done so much prep work and made everyone so twitchy. It would be anti-climatic and embarrassing to quit now.

Check-In and Pre-Op

Check-in time at the surgical center was 7:00 am. We got there with plenty of time to spare because we left at 4:30 am for an hour's drive. Crazy woman walking was still in control. I laughed my ass off when I saw it was right next to a funeral home and there was a guy outside washing his hearse. I refused to park facing the hearse; I drove clear over to the other side of the parking lot...no sense tempting the Fates before their first cup of coffee.

After check-in, I went back with a nurse to be weighed, have my blood pressure taken and wait to get set up for anesthesia. I met with the anesthesiologist. They got my IV going and gave me antibiotics and something to relax me before they did the nerve block. They wrote "yes" on the correct shoulder. I'm glad I had the nerve block, but it was really weird when they lifted my arm to test it. You would swear it was somebody else's arm next to your head...effective, but creepy.

My surgeon came in to check on me and we were good to go. I was feeling relaxed and happier than I had felt in months...my hands were up and I was flying down the roller coaster. I was wheeled into the operating room, told to breathe deeply and that was it until I woke up in recovery. I remember being thirsty and the recovery nurse holding a straw to my lips and drinking down a Coke. What I really wanted was a cup of coffee. When the nurse felt I was ready to go home, it was showtime, literally – I had to get some clothes on.

Getting Dressed to Go Home

The nurse was cool with the pajama pants (they let you keep your underpants on for shoulder surgery), but she almost had apoplexy over my oversized camisole. "Don't! You can't move your arm!" She calmed down when she realized I didn't have to move my arm and the strap was only for my good side...I just needed to raise it up far enough to cover myself on the surgery side. She strapped me into my state-of-the-art sling which had three big clips, three sets of Velcro, an abduction pillow that fit between my body and the sling, an adjustable waistband, an adjustable neck band and a nifty squeezy ball. I was still pretty loopy...you'll wish your sling had come with a DVD because you're never gonna remember how to get out of it, much less how to get back in it again!

When I single-handedly put on my one armed t-shirt and carefully arranged the side drapey part over my shoulder and sling, the nurse was impressed. "Where did you get that shirt? That's the best idea I've seen!" Preparation and practice really helped...I was suitably dressed and in the backseat of the car for the drive home, quickly and efficiently. The nerve block was doing its thing -- I was feeling no pain. We stopped at the nearest Starbucks and I ordered a grande nonfat cinnamon dolce latte, three pumps not four, with whipped cream. Time to head home!

Chapter 5:

PHASE ONE

The First Day

My family was ready and waiting for me. My caregiver locked me in the car with the keys in the ignition after we pulled into the driveway. I just looked at her and said "get the spare set because I can't help you." Good thing we had a spare set...I was as helpless as a newborn, caffeinated baby at that point. My surgery had gone well, but the anterior portion of my rotator cuff was too far retracted and frayed to repair. However, my posterior side was viable, so I had two suture anchors in that side. And two suture stitches. I didn't have any sutures in my bicep. The surgeon decided it would cause me too much pain and limited movement with no benefit.

I made it into the house supported by my son and settled into the recliner. The caregiver went off to pick up my pain meds and baby aspirin. I had to take one baby aspirin per day for two weeks to prevent blood clots. I needed to apply ice to the operated shoulder for 72 hours by applying cold packs to my shoulder for 20 minutes at a time to reduce pain and swelling. They didn't put me in a cryo cuff at the surgical center. The one I purchased was a fail because we had bought it off of Ebay and never tested it out. For some unknown reason it wouldn't work. That was a good thing because I couldn't have moved my arm and shoulder to put the damn cryo cuff on anyway and I would have hurt my repair trying! I tried a gel ice pack but that felt too heavy, so we resorted to using two bags of frozen peas and carrots – much lighter and easier to shape into position. It would take a few days to be able to stand the weight of the bigger ice pack. My arm and shoulder were still comfortably numb.

I wasn't supposed to stress my suture line, drive, smoke or take a tub bath. Fat chance of any of that happening. I wasn't going anywhere. I needed to be in the care of a responsible adult for the first 24 hours. Check. I needed to take my pain meds with a small snack and stay ahead of the pain. Check. I needed to use the restroom within eight hours. Double check. I was to keep my shoulder repair arm elevated above my heart while resting. Check. Since I was in the sling with the abduction pillow it couldn't be anywhere else. I was NOT to lift my arm at the shoulder using my muscles. Checkity check check check. You couldn't pay me to move my arm at all at that point!

When you first come home from surgery, well-meaning friends and family are going to think they can hug you. Don't let them. Be nice but let them know that's not an option. Even one arm hugs with your good arm hurt too much and put your repair arm at a weird angle. Air hugs only! There will be time for hugging in about six weeks, if then. They can wave at you, hold your good hand, kiss you gently on the forehead without touching any other part of your body, but don't let them hug you. Keep that shoulder protected and still. Your sling is usually necessary for four to six weeks for your comfort and to protect the repaired tendon.

Don't let your dog or cat jump up near your arm and shoulder area. They are worried about you; you smell like hospital. They want to let you know how much they love you. They want to give you kisses and maybe lick on that arm in that mysterious sling. Let them snuggle you on your good side but keep them away from your repair. Also, make sure that your dog who likes to herd you around the house or your cat who likes to wind around your legs is not underfoot when you get up to use the bathroom. They are well-meaning but a fall can cause real damage and there's all that money down the drain because Sweetie or Rover wanted to be close to you. Don't be a sucker for the affection. Keep them away and be in control of how close they get to you.

Removing the Dressing

The next day it was time to remove my dressing. My arm was much less numb. Removing the dressing wasn't easy. My caregiver worked slowly, but I was nervous and apprehensive which didn't make it easier. It wasn't because it was painful or anything – my pain was managed well. It was because I had no idea what to expect...and I was scared of the unknown. I imagined big black stitches over a bloody gaping wound...Walking Dead style. It was actually small and neat with a few stitches covered with steri-strips. Nothing to write home about. If I'd had a reference point of a picture or a description, I would have been more relaxed. You're not supposed to remove the steri-strips. They'll come off on their own. I was told I could shower if I covered them with waterproof band-aids or plastic wrap, but I wasn't to use or move my shoulder at all. No, thank you, I'd pass on the shower for awhile.

Whose Directions Should I Follow?

The nurse at the surgical center said to *gently* take my arm out of the sling and *gently* (big word in shoulder surgery) let my arm hang by my side to allow my elbow to straighten out a few times a day. When I saw my doctor five days later, he said, "Oh no. Don't do that. Stop doing that. Wait until physical therapy next week to start any of that." Okay. Too late, but okay. Moral of the story: you may get conflicting advice. Keep asking questions until you make sure you are doing exactly what your doctor's protocol is.

I didn't do any harm by straightening my elbow, but I did give myself an uncomfortable few days because I took the damnable sling completely off in sections and put it back on incorrectly. Remember I said it had a large abduction pillow which acted as a spacer between my body and the sling? It was beautifully designed with Velcro on one side to attach to the sling and a curved side to go against your body. Well, fear combined with pain meds and no clue of how it all went together in the first place resulted in me velcroing the sling on top of the

79

cushion and putting my bicep in a rotten cramp for about 36 hours until I couldn't take it any longer. Something didn't look right and it hurt.

I pulled up pictures of the sling in use on someone's arm on the internet and realized what I did wrong. I took it off and reconfigured it...sweet blessed relief! It is so important to make sure you know exactly how your sling is set up BEFORE you take it off. The sling I was sent home from the hospital in was the Shoulder Abduction Sling with Pillow. If you are able to find out what sling you will be sent home in, it would help. You can probably find pictures and videos on the internet to help you figure out how to take it on and off. Some are more complicated than others.

The First Few Days

Friends and family will come and visit, bringing treats and meals. You'll be pretty sedated and sleepy in your recliner chair. If you had the nerve block, during the first twenty-four to thirty-six hours your arm will slowly regain sensation. In order to keep your pain level manageable, take your pain medications exactly as prescribed at the exact times and never let the pain get ahead of you.

Notify your doctor immediately if your pain isn't under control. You can't rest and heal properly if you are in pain.

Your world will narrow and slow to a turtle crawl. Your body has a fragile part you have to baby and guard. Your shoulder repair needs to be kept as still and immobile as possible. If someone needs something, you won't be able to provide it. You have one job: guard your repair at all costs. Everything will get done, but without your constant vigilance.

The first few days you'll eat, sleep and go to the bathroom, just like a baby. Get up regularly and move slowly around your house. Walking up and down a main hallway a few times each hour helps to keep your blood flowing and your muscles moving. You don't want a blood clot. Also, make sure there are no mats or throw rugs that could trip you.

Sh*t Happens

You'll need help opening pain medication containers the first few days, especially if you have child safety caps due to children in the household. Please make sure whoever handles your medication is trustworthy. The nicest, most competent people can have addiction problems.

I learned the hard way. I had to let my caregiver go after the first four days. I have kept any and all pain medications locked up since. I should have done it to begin with, I should have only trusted my husband, I should have counted them every time...but I didn't. Sometimes people position themselves to be caregivers so they have easier access to pain medications. You're probably more savvy than I am but for what it's worth, be wary of who you place in charge of your pain meds during those first few days when you can't open the container yourself.

Here it was Day 5. I had let my caregiver go. I didn't know how or what I was going to feed my family for dinner. I had to be at my first doctor's check-up in Little Rock the next day and I had just fired my ride! That take-charge woman who had everything under control? She was long gone; disappeared into a cloud of anesthesia. Sometimes it all has to fall apart before a new, better something can rise up -- better than what I could have planned. Because it wasn't my plan...it was a collaborative effort of friends and family who stepped in and helped this shaky control freak breathe and lean on them for support.

You'll find if you just ask, people will help. You'll get that ride to the doctor's office. You'll have dinner that night delivered by a friend. You will make it through that day and the next one and the next. Just keep breathing. Even when you are uncomfortable, hurting and wanting to lash out at someone in frustration, keep breathing.

Day 6 arrived, grey and stormy with thunder and lightening. I hadn't slept well. I felt like a cat whose fur had been brushed the wrong way. I was jumpy and wanted to bite someone. I didn't know how I was going to navigate wet stairs, water puddles and climbing into the backseat of the car with my pillow to support my arm and my blanket so I wouldn't freeze in my t-shirt poncho. Getting dressed, using the bathroom and brushing my teeth took a long time. I kept sitting down to rest. My husband came in and said, "Still working on the underpants? You go, girl." and left for the office. My hero.

First Doctor Appointment After the Surgery

This was a tough appointment. I was nervous and not prepared for the looks I got in the doctor's office. The waiting room holds about forty patients on a regular day and it was filled. No one was wearing post surgical garb like mine. I looked like hell. In a wilted t-shirt poncho. With spiky baby chicken warrior hair. Even the nurse wasn't sure what to do with my new look. I think the open air side was freaking everyone out. Even when he checked my stitches, he kept re-draping it. Like my boobs were going to magically appear in some uncontained fashion. I had this; I was completely, if unconventionally, covered.

The nurse will check your incision site, front and back. Mine was fine. He'll tell you that the surgical strips will come off in the shower on their own and give you orders for when to start physical therapy. Until my physical therapy evaluation, I wasn't to move my shoulder. The doctor would see me again in six weeks. I was to keep squeezing the squeezy ball that my right hand rested on at the end of my sling. It helped my circulation and kept my hand from freezing in one position. I was also to keep icing every 15-20 minutes as needed which would help with pain.

During Phase One your surgeon has specific goals. These goals are to protect your repair, make sure your wound is healing properly, prevent your shoulder from stiffening up and help you regain your passive range of motion during the first six weeks of recovery. You can use the hand on your repair arm, but you can't lift your arm or elbow away from your body. Don't lift anything with your repair arm no matter how small. Don't extend or make sudden movements with your shoulder and don't support your body weight with your hands at all for any reason.

Sex and Your Shoulder Surgery

Face it. It's awkward. If you even feel like having sex during the first six weeks, you'll have to be creative. By about the third or fourth week, you may feel brave enough to try. Keep your sling on and don't let your shoulder move. Not the most erotic, but it works. Also, your partner will have to understand you can only be the beneficiary in this romantic interlude. Any attempt to reciprocate can result in pain. Remember? No supporting of your body weight with your hands. Also, keep it mellow, nice and easy. Any sudden moves will hurt and distract you from the moment. Keep it light, keep it fun and enjoy the closeness. All those good endorphins fizzing through your bloodstream after orgasm can help reduce your pain, induce relaxation and put you in a good mood -- great for when you're down in the dumps and singing the "I'm stuck in a sling and can't move after surgery" blues.

Handicapped Stalls in Restrooms

Use them! When you're at the doctor's office and you have to use the restroom, use the handicapped stall. It's one thing to use the bathroom at home; it's another to use one when you are away from home. Everything is a different height and unfamiliar. The handicapped stall is big enough for you to maneuver around in with your sling so you don't hit the sides of the stall or the toilet paper holder. Plus, use the bar to hang onto with your good hand so you don't lose your balance and fall over. There are also enough hooks to hold whatever you are carrying. This is not the time to carry the tiny designer handbag. A good, sturdy bag with handles that can fit all your paperwork, appointment cards, cell phone, pain meds, snacks and a water bottle is better.

Anxiety and the Blues

The next few days were rocky. I tried to figure out what to do with myself. I did mini laps up and down my hallway. I called the doctor's nurse concerned about my surgical strips, whether I had hurt my shoulder because I had been startled during a scary part in a movie, could I hypothetically do damage to my repair if I moved the wrong way in my sleep? He answered all my questions, reassuring me the best he could, and finally said "You know, Mrs. Cooksey, it might not be a bad idea to think about taking some anxiety medicine." Back to breathing.

After you're home for about a week it begins to sink in that you've really gone and had shoulder surgery. And you are in this sling for six long weeks. That revelation is tough. The bloom is off the rose. Visitors and phone calls have slowed down. You don't want to read another book or watch another movie and the children want to know why you can't drive them to Walmart to look at action figures. Don't freak out if you find yourself really, really depressed and sad. It's the aftermath of all the months of anxious decision-making and preparations, after effects of the anesthesia, your body feeling violated and in pain, the irrefutable fact that you are stuck in this sling and your arm bloody hurts! Have a good, long cry with a big box of tissues. Crying is good for the body and soul. Crying releases pent-up emotions and stress. Shoulder surgery is a means to an end. You want your arm to work properly and stop hurting on a daily basis. But it's also frustrating, overwhelming and painful. That's a good reason to sob it all out. When the storm passes, hang on to the knowledge that it's not forever. Someday in the future you'll be back to your old activities and cruising the aisles of Walmart picking up tennis balls for your Saturday tennis match. Yes, you will.

One week after my surgery, I lost it. I was frustrated, slow, unwashed and feeling oh so sorry for myself. I simply would not, could not last six more weeks in this horrible sling. My family was out doing whatever they did on Saturdays. I had an all-out crying session, loud and ugly with snot streaming down my face and big boo-hoo-hoo tears. My dog hid in the closet. When I was done, I blew my nose, wiped my eyes and gave myself a piece of my own mind. It was only for six weeks. Time to live up to my warrior hairdo and get back on the positivity train.

I made a list of what I could do:

1. Make a daily To Do chart with big check-off boxes
2. Make a Giant Six Week Calendar and stick it up on the wall
3. Sing 3 Karaoke songs standing in front of the computer each day
4. Take a shower -- baby wipes weren't cutting it
5. Go on a daily walk outside in the sun

To-Do Chart:

After the first week, your days start to blend into one another. You go mad without any activities to occupy your time. One way to give your day some shape is to make up a To-Do List/Check-off Chart. People make lists for a reason; it gives a sense of accomplishment to check things off. It's even more of a rush if you get to put your check mark in a box. It's totally psychological. You can put things on it like "went to the bathroom without help" with ten boxes to check off, "meals" with three boxes, "Vitamins" with one box or more depending how many times a day you take them. You can put "nap" on there with as many check off boxes you want! It's just a visual so you can see what you got done that day. If you're having free-floating anxiety or feeling sad, useless and in pain, you can "pet the dog" and check off a box or two. It gives you some choices, helps you remember to eat and take your meds and makes you feel good. You'll find yourself making up categories to put on there so you can check off more boxes.

Goal and Milestone Calendar:

Make a big two-month paper calendar and put all your goals and milestones on it. Your first post-surgery doctor visit, your first shower, your physical therapy evaluation, your first real t-shirt with sides, your second post-surgery doctor visit, and of course, the exact six week date. That magic date when you will, hopefully, get to take the sling off. Checking off each completed day makes you feel you are making progress – even if your progress is just that big black Sharpie X on the calendar. When you are feeling slap-crappy, look at how far you have come. Keep a journal. If you can't write, use your phone's notepad feature and built-in microphone. Email it to yourself to paste into a document. When you are at week three and your hair is washed and you are sufficiently medicated, throw yourself a party. Put it on your calendar. Call everybody you know, tell them to bring something to share, including ice and beverages, and have them all gather around your recliner and say nice things about you. Oh, do it. You know you want to. You have to strike when the iron is hot and everyone feels your pain. They won't be so lapdoggy when you are huffing around on your own two feet again. Enjoy it while you can!

Singing:

Singing does help. You don't need to sound like an American Idol contestant. You don't have to sound good at all. It's all about relieving emotion and pent-up stress.

Like a burst of laughter, singing helps clear away the depression cobwebs and creates happy space in your brain. Stand in front of the computer so you can get some air into your diaphragm, go to YouTube and choose your favorite karaoke songs. No one's listening, so belt them out! Sing three songs and go check them off. You may find you simultaneously sing and cry at the same time for a few days. I did. My boys would just look at me crying and singing, shake their heads and walk away. Music is powerful stuff. Singing is a lot of toning which is used in many healing therapies. Whatever the reason, it was the right, intuitive way to deal with my frustration and depression. After I sang out all those tears, they never returned.

Go for a Walk:

Keep your mood elevated with a short, daily walk down the street. Get those leg muscles moving and oxygen flowing through your blood – more positive healing energy. Stitch together as many ragged pieces of your courage as you can and walk down the driveway. You will need to have another person with you to hang on to, literally. Walk with someone who is calm, patient, protective and attentive. This is not to get your heart rate up. This is an airing, a stroll. It takes a kind person and strong self esteem to walk carefully, arm in arm, with a shuffling, nervous mother dressed like a hobo in a giant sling, clutching at them and squawking "Hold on tight! Don't let me fall! Don't go so fast!" over and over like an ADHD parrot. If you are up to it, it's nice to be outside walking. Choose a day that's dry and sunny. Any sort of wet weather leads to slippery conditions which are not advised. It will feel so normal. All you need to do is keep your repair safe from harm and hang on to your sturdy companion with your good arm. Enjoy your walk; it's just enough of a break in the monotony to keep the bats out of the belfry.

Help, I Need Somebody!

"People, people who need people...are the luckiest people in the world." Cue the Barbra Streisand music and swallow your pride. Even though your shoulder is in a sling and your rear end is confined to your recliner most of the day, you have a phone and a voice -- USE THEM! It may be the only exercise you get for a while...let those fingers do the walking and ask people for help. Most people want to help, they just need a specific task to do. If you need a meal prepared and delivered, a ride to the doctor's office, medicine picked up or a load of laundry washed and folded, ASK! You can always repay the favor someday or pay it forward to someone else. I depended on the kindness of friends and strangers alike because my pride was gone, along with my hair and my ability to take off my socks. Life gets very basic, very quickly. I promise you -- it gets easier the more you practice. "Please?" and "thank you" accomplish miracles.

Children are helpful little critters and like to be part of your recovery. Give them things to do like unload the dishwasher and find your glasses. It makes them feel less anxious. They're not used to seeing you trussed up like a mummy in your recliner or crawling down the hall like a Heinz Ketchup drip to go to the bathroom. This is a huge disruption in their schedule. Children do well with routine and security. When a parent has surgery, the whole household starts slinking around like startled cats. Try to prepare them beforehand, make charts of simple chores and daily activities. Keep their morning and evening routine the same as best you can for consistency. By the afternoon, the day may lose structure and dissolve into a massive free for all of Cheetos, television and video games. When the 5:00 pm witching hour strikes, a schedule will help them come to their senses and head into the evening routine.

As you get into a daily routine, be protective of yourself. Move gingerly. Be aware of your body. Pain is your best indicator. You won't want to move in any direction or do anything that would make it more uncomfortable than it already is. We're used to throwing our bodies around and making them work really hard. We stretch them in the wrong direction, hoping they'll just snap back so we can keep going. For right now, accept your limitations because the body doesn't always snap back...sometimes it just snaps.

Physical Therapy Evaluation

My physical therapy evaluation was scheduled at 9:15 am on Day 14. I slunk into the big, bright physical therapy room with a defeated air of great weakness and fragility. "Hi, Mrs. Cooksey! Take off your sling and step over here so we can get your arm moving!" The only words I computed were "take off your sling." I ignored "arm moving" completely. "What?!" "How?!" I didn't have a clue how to take off my sling. I had unbuckled the top shoulder strap once a day to let my arm rest naturally, supported by a pillow. Other than that, the sling and I were one. Taking it off would be like unzipping my skin and stepping out of it. The sling was my security blanket.

It was put on by the surgical people; it would have to be surgically removed. "Ha-ha!" laughed my physical therapist. "Take off the sling." She ended up having to help me out of it while I breathed and tried not to embarrass myself by bursting into tears. The only thing I remember from that first day was acute fear coupled with the sheer amazement of straightening my arm and letting it hang down while doing these little circles with it, clockwise and counterclockwise.

Physical Therapy Is Not for Wimps

Your physical therapist is your best buddy. She knows exactly how much you can do, how much is too much and where you need to be with your passive and active range of motion. She is rooting for you to succeed and go back to tennis, golfing, weight-lifting or, in my case, playing guitar. She is brutally honest and does not pander to your perceived frailty. She is coach, cheerleader and teammate all rolled up into one. Trust is key. You have to get to a point of absolute faith and trust in your physical therapist. Your repair is literally in her hands and stretching out those unused muscles is gonna hurt. Not in a bad way, but in a "let's get this arm moving again the way it's supposed to!" way. The first time you are asked to remove your sling, it will be daunting. Yes, you hate the thing, but in terms of security, it's the only thing standing between you and your arm falling off. You'll start out with the mildest range of motion exercises. Not only will you be astonished you can accomplish these, you will be shocked that you are without your sling for a full 45 minutes. When you are all done, you get to sit in a chair with muscle stimulation pads attached to your shoulder while you enjoy a huge ice pack which feels so good. As time goes on and you move through the different stages, you will have more exercises added using bands, weights and other tools to increase both your strength and your range of motion.

I went to Physical Therapy three times a week. I had three sets of exercises to do daily. These were passive range of motion exercises that took about ten minutes each set. Each set had to be done while my arm was out of the sling, which created a lot of anxiety in the beginning for all of us. After I removed my sling in the bedroom, I would walk down the hall to the kitchen/laundry room area where I did my exercises, intoning in a loud voice, "Vulnerable! I am Vulnerable! Vulnerable! I am Vulnerable!" This was meant to clear the decks and get everyone out of my way. It drove my family batty and made the dog leap around my legs thinking this was a new way of saying "Let's go in the car!"

I was obsessive about my exercises. I put them on my Daily To Do list with three big boxes to check off. I'm first-rate at following directions. If you explain to me what muscle I am strengthening, what is happening inside and NO, I AM NOT HURTING MY REPAIR IN ANY WAY SHAPE OR FORM, I am devoted to doing them to the best of my ability. All the physical therapists (one wasn't enough) had to keep reassuring me that these range of motion exercises were not harmful. It was more harmful if I didn't move. I had a bad habit of keeping my arm in a protective sling position, even when my sling was off, while I walked around the therapy room. "Put your arm down, Mrs. Cooksey." "Relax your arm down, Mrs. Cooksey." "Mrs. Cooksey, PUT THE ARM DOWN!"

I was not very good at following directions when it came time for my physical therapist to stretch my arm and manipulate it manually. "You're not relaxing and giving me your arm, Mrs. Cooksey." "I don't want to, it hurts." "Did you take your pain medication?" "No." "Why not?" "If I did, I wouldn't be able to tell if you were hurting me." That's when she explained, while she didn't advocate taking pain medication if I didn't need it, I really needed to take my prescribed pain medication before physical therapy. Otherwise I wouldn't relax enough to allow her to work with my arm. I would still be able to say "ouch" if necessary, but I wouldn't be so tense and in pain to begin with. I decided to take her advice. I also decided to take the surgical nurse's advice and get a prescription for anxiety medication, too. Everybody needs to do what is right for them. I needed to relax and give over the reins if I was going to progress.

Before Your Physical Therapy Session

Start getting ready for your physical therapy sessions early. Give yourself enough time to wash and dress before you have to leave. Make sure you are reasonably clean. Put on fresh clothes and deodorant so you don't smell. When you can't raise your arm to shave or air out your armpit, it can get pretty rank. Make sure your clothing is securely in place because you will be a-movin' and a-swingin' and you don't want to flash anyone. As you build up confidence in taking off your sling, you may be ready for a button-up shirt or a loose t-shirt with both sides intact. I was now a pro at taking off my sling. Instead of a t-shirt drape, I graduated to my husband's short-sleeve button-up shirts. With my short, short hair, my button-up shirt and my sensible shoes, my youngest son said I looked like "Ellen." Not glamorous, Maybelline

CoverGirl Ellen, but still...huge compliment. He adored Ellen. Which meant he adored me. That helped.

Phase One Exercises

Be a pro-active fanatic when it comes to your shoulder exercises. Everything I could get my hands on to read emphasized how important it was to a complete recovery to do these exercises religiously. I was on it! Three times a day I marched into the laundry room and did my Phase One routine, working up from 15 repetitions to 30 repetitions over time.

1. let arm hang relaxed straight down; gently swing back and forth 30X
2. let arm hang relaxed straight down; gently swing side to side 30X
3. let arm hang relaxed straight down; gentle circles clockwise 30X
4. let arm hang relaxed straight down; gentle circles counterclockwise 30X
5. shoulder shrugs 30x
6. shoulder squeezes 30x
7. bicep curls/elbow straightens 15X
8. step-backs 30X

9. arm supported wrist to elbow, rotate body away to a gentle stretch holding 5-10 seconds for 30X

I was able to do the bicep curls because I didn't have any bicep involvement in my surgery. That was a plus for me. You may not have that ability yet. Your physical therapist will give you the exact exercises you need based on your particular surgeon and what your surgery entailed. During my physical therapy sessions, she would put me in the passive range of motion machines. I liked the machines because I felt they were predictable. The machine wouldn't go farther than the set measurement. I would always try to top my last measurement. My difficulty came in letting go and giving the physical therapist free rein to work on my range of motion. That was harder because I had a lot of tenderness in my shoulder capsule area. I used to close my eyes and pretend I was in the machine. Or in a space ship being tortured by aliens.

Handicapped Doors -- Use Them!

Most places are equipped with handicapped doors. Push the big button that has a picture of a wheelchair on it and watch the doors open. Sometimes there's two sets of double doors. There can be a circle button to the side of the door or there can be a smaller, rectangular button on a post. This is the best way to get into a building when you are by yourself. Unless you have a companion with you, don't try to open any doors by yourself. Usually the doors with the handicap buttons are heavy. These doors can close on you or clip the back of your heel. When you have only one arm, they can be dangerous. One drawback with these doors is that sometimes they stop working. Sometimes they malfunction or the electricity goes out. If the office building closes at 6:00 pm and you don't get out of your physical therapy appointment until 6:10 pm, the automatic button function may be turned off. At this point call someone for help. The doors will always work manually but you will need someone to open the door and help you out of the building. When you are recovering from surgery, watch out for building maintenance such as floors being washed in front of the handicapped doors or the restrooms. Wet floors are slippery. You can fall and undo your repair. Any time you are in an office building, a grocery store or a doctor's office, be aware of the maintenance people doing their routine cleaning of the building.

Chapter 6:

PHASE TWO

Second Doctor Appointment

Phase Two is six to twelve weeks after surgery. The surgeon's goals are to continue to protect your repair, continue to improve your range of motion and begin light strengthening. I was psyched for my second doctor's appointment. I had my physical therapy report, I was in a button-up shirt and I was hoping to be told I could lose the sling. Lots of people get overwhelmed during doctor appointments. There's so much information to take in: discussions about your progress and what the next steps are. It's easy to forget to ask some of your questions. Type up every question you can possibly think of. Print them out and bring them with you because you're going to kick yourself if you forget to ask all of them.

Here are my second appointment questions:

1. Step backs: yes, feel stretch underneath, also burning & slight stabby pressure on top. Am I doing something wrong?

2. After step backs and turnouts, (doing one extra set per day to open up exterior rotation), same burn/stabby pain on top. If that's okay, then I'll keep going, but I don't know what is a "stop, too much" pain indicator.

3. Hand really stiff and painful in morning; what is correct sleeping position?

4. Odd times during day/night: medieval dance party with stabbing localized pain. Normal healing?

5. Bend over to pick something up with good hand; feel dull pressure/pain in repair area. Normal?

6. Really hard time relaxing with manual prom by therapist. Hard time trusting. Now take full pain meds before therapy and anxiety meds. Relaxed more and got better range of motion. Still fighting therapist a bit no matter how hard I try to psyche myself out and relax. Normal?

7. Still using pain meds/ice packs. Heat?

8. Sling off soon?

9. Driving?

10. When can I lie down in bed?

11. Please take off steri-strips?

The nurse asked me to take off my sling. He checked my range of motion. He said I was done with the sling. He took my question sheet and read them all carefully. He answered each question fully and to my satisfaction. Despite all the showers I had been taking, my surgical steri-strips were still hanging on. They were supposed to have fallen off in the shower, but mine were not budging. I was too scared to pull them off myself because I didn't want any shoulder guts to fall out. When he got to #11, he looked at my shoulder and gently took them off without a word. Ahhhh, relief. He also let me know that I would be feeling lots of inexplicable sensations in my shoulder as things healed. Unless the pain was constant and increasing, I wasn't to worry. He said driving would have to wait until my range of motion allowed me to have both hands on the wheel in the 10 and 2 position easily.

I saw the surgeon who checked my shoulder carefully, ordered more physical therapy and waved me through to the second six weeks of Phase Two. First six weeks done! 42 sharpie X's on the calendar marked off! I was really excited to get to work on increasing my range of motion so I could drive.

Figuring Out Your Limitations in Phase Two

During the second six weeks you'll begin to get a little careless. Don't feel bad. We all do. You'll get cocky. You're driving. You're gaining more range of motion. You think, "I can lift this full trash bag out of the kitchen trashcan; I can sort of pick up this container of milk if I balance it against my good arm for support." You'll sit down and use both hands to play the piano right after you've done your set of exercises. You'll make a bed and tuck the bottom sheet in. You'll fold the laundry with two hands and maybe shake the shirt a little too hard or move your arm a little too wide. You really aren't doing anything that will damage your repair but now you're feeling achy and a bit strained. That happens. It's almost as if you have to overdo to figure out your limitations and realize "ouch! I can't do that." At that point, drag out your ice pack, go sit in a chair and rest. Be nice to yourself about it. Don't kick yourself or think "I'm a failure. I've put my recovery back and I'm a disappointment to everyone who is rooting for me." You'll get over it. You'll be back in your routine and think twice before you reach for something, overextend or do something when you're tired.

When Did I Last Eat Something?

Yes, it's important to care about what sort of shape you are in before you have elective surgery. Yes, it's important to attempt to maintain a healthy diet before surgery to enable the best possible healing. After shoulder surgery is a different story. For the first couple of weeks you will eat whatever people put in front of you because you can't get it for yourself. Eat something to protect your stomach from the pain medications. Sometimes all you can reach with your good hand is the bag of cookies the kids left near your chair. Until you are able to fix your own food or supervise the shopping again, go with the flow.

The weeks went by and I started eating very healthily. I knew protein was necessary for building strong muscles and tendons. Well, I was in the process of growing a baby supraspinatus. I ate leafy, green vegetables and chugged protein powder smoothies. I dutifully checked off my healthy meals on my To Do chart. After a few weeks of healthy eating and daily walking in the neighborhood, I was feeling good. I'd even lost five lbs. I was back to doing some paperwork at home for the office. Then I started putting off lunch later and later in the day. My husband came home from work to find me sitting at the dining room table surrounded by dozens of folders of paperwork. It was around 2:00 pm. I looked up at him and said "I feel weird." Then, "I think I'm blacking out." He rushed over to me, made me put my head down and said right away, "what did you eat today?" "Nothing, just my vitamins." He ran to the kitchen, poured me a big glass of orange juice, got me a banana and made me eat it. "Do you realize if I hadn't come home at this very minute you would have passed out, crashed to the floor and injured your shoulder again??" "Yes," I said, stuffing the banana in my mouth as fast as I could. "Don't ever do that again; you have to eat! You just had surgery!"

Keep Your Energy Up

I don't care if you can't tell the difference between an eggplant or a dingdong, just make sure you eat something. If you don't eat, you get weak. If you get weak, you get dizzy. If you get dizzy, you fall down. Don't do what I did. Make good choices. Your shoulder is repairing at this time. Eat as healthily as you can but make sure you are getting enough food into you. That means if your only choice is a strawberry frosted PopTart or nothing, eat the damned PopTart. You'll know when you need to cut back. That unpleasant feeling when your yoga pants feel like yoga Spanx? More fruit and veggies, less Hershey's Miniatures. It's a balance.

During Phase One and Phase Two of your shoulder surgery recovery, it's a great idea to have a little portable survival kit. It can include a water bottle, a juice box, some cheese, some dried fruit and nuts and maybe a granola bar or a candy bar. Add some tissues, some antibacterial wipes, some baby wipes and a few band aids – you will be very popular wherever you go. Take it with you whenever you leave the house for a doctor's appointment or physical therapy. It's rotten being stranded somewhere if your ride is running late and you don't have something to eat or drink. You can get tired and squirrelly after these appointments. It might have been several hours since you ate anything. You feel like you're going to faint...oh crap...then you realize that in your bag you tucked a granola bar, a box of raisins and a water bottle. Yeah, you just saved your own day. You are probably thinking "I am a grown up. I don't need to be reminded about these things." Guess what? After shoulder surgery, all that puffy arrogance goes out the window with your remaining brain cells. You hurt. Your concentration is shot because you are trying to make sure you stay upright and you don't walk into something by accident. Been there, done that, got the bruise. It's good to have a little survival kit so you don't go all horizontal and kiss the floor.

I was at a doctor's appointment, bone tired and loopy from getting dressed. It had been hours since I had breakfast. I was so dizzy I thought, "Oh jeez, I'm going down." There was a little coffee area, but no coffee. I poured sugar packets into a styrofoam coffee cup, mixed them with drinking fountain water and sucked it all down. I didn't have any snacks in my bag which was a really dumb move on my part. I knew better. I never left the house again without my survival kit.

Yoga

Yoga is a great exercise because there are so many different levels. When you begin your yoga at about month four or five, it isn't a big deal. Put in your yoga DVD or pull up one that is for beginners on Gaiam TV. Watch it. Wave at your feet to let them know you're thinking about them. I especially like the yoga DVDs with a beautiful ocean in the background. I like to listen to the instructor's soothing voice, watch the water, listen to the relaxing music and take a nap. Be realistic. You can't do exactly what the yoga instructor is doing because you can't move your arm in that direction. You may not even be able to get down on the floor yet. Or if you do get down on the floor, there's no way in hell you're going to get back up. It takes time. Yoga is a great exercise for people who like or need to take a lot of time.

Stress Relief Yoga for Beginners by Suzanne Deason is a 22-minute relaxation yoga routine. You can purchase it on Amazon and it's available with a Gaiam TV subscription. This isn't one of those kundalini fire pillar, build your core, burn baby burn yoga programs. This is a program to reduce stress and deeply relax. Relaxation yoga is my favorite. It involves a lot of deep breathing and stretching. It's not only your shoulder muscles that have been out of commission. It's also your back muscles, your leg muscles, your hip muscles – pretty much every muscle on your body has been in hibernation during Phase One and Phase Two of your shoulder repair recovery. Yoga is a nice way to wake them up without startling them.

You can begin Stress Relief Yoga at any level of physical ability. If all you can do that particular day is lay down on your yoga mat, listen to her voice and enjoy the swish of the ocean waves in the background, so be it.

Many times my husband walked into the living room while I was on my yoga mat, flat on my back with my dog curled up in my armpit. "I thought you were doing yoga." "I am doing yoga." "That's a funny kind of yoga. You look like you're sleeping with Fluffy." "I'm working up to it, dear." If you can't move your arm yet but you can sit on the floor, it shows you how to stretch out your legs and hips. I've had problems with restless leg syndrome during recovery, so I try to keep my legs and hips stretched out. Otherwise, I end up all hitchy and crinkled. Angry, achy legs when you're in a big pillow sling are not fun.

Walking

In Phase Two you'll be ready to walk by yourself next to somebody without holding onto their arm. At this point it's helpful to use a cane or walking stick. Even though there's nothing wrong with your legs, you're weaker than you realize. Using a walking stick in your good hand gives you more stability. After you build up your legs and you're confident using your walking stick, you'll be able to walk by yourself down the street without a companion. Walking with some sort of assistance when you are on an uneven surface like a neighborhood road or sidewalk will help you guard against tripping and falling. Your repair is being held in place by sutures. If you fall, those sutures can cut right through that muscle and tendon and sever the repair. Baby yourself. By your third or fourth month you'll be able to walk without a support. You'll even be able to walk the dog again. Still, you need to be aware and watch where you're going. Leave yourself enough time for your scheduled walk. Rushing and hurrying are the antithesis of a successful recovery from shoulder surgery.

Even six months into recovery you need to be aware and careful while walking. I was walking our dog, Fluffy, at night with my husband. Fluffy spied an armadillo munching on bugs in a neighbor's yard. Fluffy went wild and launched himself at the armadillo. At the same time, a small herd of twelve deer leaped across the road. Our small dog started to spin around me in circles, winding me up in the leash. I stepped on Fluffy. He yelped. John grabbed the leash and stepped on Fluffy. Fluffy yelped louder. John flinched and grabbed my repair arm so we wouldn't fall down. He didn't grab too hard and let go right away because I screeched "SHOULDER!" I was fine, but it could have ended differently. If he had fallen and yanked me down by my repaired shoulder or if I had fallen and taken the brunt of the fall on my repaired shoulder, I could have done major damage. That's how fast I could have undone all my hard work because I was too busy laughing at the chaos and not aware of my surroundings.

A Tiny Bit of Laundry

When you are in Phase Two of your recovery, you will be so ready to do something that folding laundry will start to look like fun. Running a load of wash that consists of one or two outfits is a good start. Sitting on the bed and folding them with your good hand for five minutes at a time is a way to feel productive again. If your physical therapist is game, you can start incorporating your repair arm. It's a light activity that helps you feel independent again. That's important. It's the little things, the baby steps.

You're not trying to take over doing the laundry again. You never want to take over the laundry again! You're just using the folding aspect of laundry as a rehabilitative exercise and a meditative motion to move your body and calm your mind at the same time. Have someone wash and dry a few clothes, then dump them on your bed. Take one item at a time, lay it down on the bed and fold it with your good hand. A towel is a good item to start with because it's just a big rectangle. It's not hard to fold corner to corner. No fitted sheets – that's a production with two good hands! When you're finished and you see a tiny lopsided pile of badly folded clothes, you'll feel proud. You accomplished something! Not a very big something and not a very hard something, but you did it! It makes sitting back down in the recliner feel like a reward and not a life sentence. It allows you to use up a little bit of your anxious energy and focus it in a productive way.

Fun With Physical Therapy

Make physical therapy sessions fun. Yup, you heard me. Get all the complaining and moaning out of your system by week three. Yes, you still hurt. Getting your range of motion back is super hard, uncomfortable work. But that doesn't mean you can't amuse yourself along the way. You can't drive anywhere by yourself. You're still stuck at home to rest and repair. But you get to be chauffeured to physical therapy at least three times a week. Okay, then. Why did you have this surgery? Are you an athlete? A musician? Did your messed up shoulder affect how you earned your living? A physical therapy room is full of exercise balls, bands and weights in bright colors, state-of-the-art equipment to get you back in gear and energetic therapists who want the best for you! How's that for a positive environment? It's your

own Disney playground for the next six months or so --
make it entertaining.

If you're looking longingly at your tennis racket
gathering dust at your front door or your favorite golf club
lying abandoned on the garage floor, bring them into
therapy. Talk to your physical therapist about what you
hope to be able to do in the future and see if they can
incorporate your racket or club into your exercise routine
at home. They aren't going to give you something that
will hurt you or you aren't ready for yet, but it's comforting
to see the light at the end of the tunnel and to start
looking forward to what you can do. Using a Star Wars
lightsaber that lights up and makes swooshy noises
instead of a plain baton at therapy can bring a smile to
your face and even encourage you to work a little harder.
Ask if you could use your racket or golf club the same
way. Having familiar items in your routine is comforting
and helps you remember this is just temporary.

Don't Settle...Get Excited

If you are longing to shampoo with two hands instead
of just one or if you are having trouble getting your arms
up to the ten and two position so you can drive again,
ask your physical therapist for help. Don't just sit there

like a mute cow doing your exercises with an air of resignation. You're paying for this; get the most out of it for maximum efficiency. Find out your limitations and what can be accomplished within them. Find out what is the six-week goal; what is the twelve-week goal. Get excited! Use this time to learn as much as you can about your shoulder and how it works and how you can devise ways to make it work even better now that it has been repaired. Don't settle for the status quo...ask about different pieces of equipment and what they are used for. Ask when you will be able to use them. Use your time there to increase your knowledge. If an exercise is difficult, ask if it can be modified so you can get the same benefit but in a different way that doesn't cause stress to your repair.

Physical therapists are in the business of getting bodies back into top-physical working condition and back on the road. You may not realize it at first when you stumble in feeling like fresh roadkill, but they're your ticket to cutting edge exercises, therapies and technologies. If you play the piano, ask how soon you can begin practicing with one hand, then with two and for how long. Once healing is underway, moving your body is necessary so you don't freeze up. When you hurt, the last thing you want to do is move the hurty part. You feel afraid you might mess up your repair if you go too fast.

That's what your physical therapist is there for – to push you to do what you can do and to hold you back until you're ready to go ahead. They won't push you beyond your capability. Now, what you *think* you are capable of and what your physical therapist *knows* you are capable of are two completely different boxes of cereal in the fun pack.

Own It, Baby!

Physical therapy is hard work. Don't freak out if you grunt, fart, ooof, or let loose a curse or two. Don't take yourself too seriously. You wouldn't be in physical therapy if you weren't ready for it. Make the most of your time and *be* on time! You'll get much more out of your therapy if you arrive early and are ready to go. As you get more comfortable with your routine, start owning your presence there. Think of it as a very exclusive private club with great perks. Don't come late and have to be prodded to begin your routine. That's bad form. When you finish one set of exercises, go on to the next one if you know what's next and surprise your therapist with your "take charge, I can do this" attitude. Some days will be harder than others. When that happens, let them know what's going on. Maybe you overdid your exercises at home; maybe you lifted the spaghetti pot before you were ready. Keep an open dialogue going with your physical therapist. They can't help you to be at your best if you don't update them on a regular basis. This is YOUR appointment. This is YOUR time to shine. Jazz hands, people, jazz hands!

New exercises will be added to your routine until you are up to roughly 20 minutes of exercises three times a day. There are different levels of resistance bands: yellow, red, green, blue. There are over-the-door pulley systems. Keep track of all your different exercises. Don't leave your therapy appointment without getting a sheet of them or writing them down. Name them things that sound like the exercises look: "Stayin' Alive", "Hoist Yer Sword, Matey", "Target Practice", "Window Washer", "Itsy Bitsy Spider", "Wax On, Wax Off." You think you'll remember all of them. You won't. You'll forget as soon as you walk out the door because you've been iced down, your pain meds have kicked in and you are feeling good. Get them down on paper.

Think you can get away with not doing your exercises at home? You just do them at your appointment and think no one will be the wiser? News Flash: Your physical therapist knows. Your physical therapist can tell by your sense of ease with the exercises, your ability to remember them in the order you were given them and by subtle changes in your muscles if you've been doing your work. You're only cheating yourself if you neglect your exercises. Your physical therapist can only help you to the extent you are willing to help yourself.

Designated Drivers

For as long as you need your pain meds for physical therapy, have someone drive you to your session. You might think you can tough it out, drive yourself and take your meds when you get home, but that's just stupid. You won't be getting all you can out of your therapy. You'll be mad and cranky when you get home and your shoulder will hurt because you didn't keep up with the pain. Be schlepped back and forth for as long as you can! Take the help. Take all of it and then, take some more. No one thinks any less of you for asking. They don't want you to push yourself and be in pain. It makes them feel good to help you. We're on this planet to be a blessing to others. Do your part and help them fill their quota. When you are completely recovered, you can do the same for someone else. You'll want to because you'll remember how hard it was to ask for help when *you* needed it.

Pain Management

Pain management is a big issue. Keep a close and open relationship with your surgeon so you get the pain medication in the dosage that you need. It's an individual thing. Some people do fine with less and some people need the maximum amount. You may have a nerve block that will help with the amount of pain you feel in the first day or so. Your arm will be completely numb. It'll feel uber funky -- like it doesn't belong to you. But having no feeling is preferable to lots of pain. Don't try to tough out your pain and take less medication then you need. Pain is debilitating. It can rob you of your energy and your happy feelings which can delay your recovery.

Try not to get down on yourself if it's the sixth week and you still need your pain medication. Everyone is different. Don't judge yourself by Joe the Jock who threw his bottle of pain medication away after the first week and hiked the Rocky Mountains in his sling with only an energy bar and a hammock. What's important is for you to listen to your body and make sure you're comfortable. Pain medication won't take away all of the pain but it will make your level of pain tolerable. If pain medication took away all the pain, we would do dumb things like using our arm when we shouldn't because heck, it doesn't hurt

-- why not go play tennis?

Be honest with yourself about your pain medication. If you need it, take it. It's a balance. You may find you don't need it as much as you progress in your therapy. Cutting back doesn't mean stopping. It means cutting back to a lower dosage. Talk to your doctor about this. If you just cut a pain pill in half, you may not be getting the dosage of Tylenol you need. There are lower dosages of pain medication that maintain the same level of Tylenol. You are not in this alone. Your doctor is your partner in monitoring your pain.

Meloxicam is an anti-inflammatory medication that is an alternative to ibuprofen. Lots of people do very well on Meloxicam. Some people can have severe, life-threatening allergic reactions, especially if they have asthma. I did. Make sure, if you are prescribed this, that you inform your doctor about all medications you are taking and what other physical issues you have.

Are you afraid you can do damage to your repair by a jumbo sneeze or doing a few more repetitions with the exercise band? A twinge or fleeting sparkle pain or the feeling a mariachi band is playing a tune inside your bicep is not cause for alarm. If something increases in severity or continues for days because you picked something up that's too heavy and the pain caused you to fall to your knees, that's bad. You probably did something. But otherwise, there's a lot of healing and reconfiguring and repairing going on inside your shoulder. Don't get all worried brow over it. Keep the ice going. Ice is your friend. Keep lots of gel cold packs in your freezer so you can rotate them. After 5:00 pm each day when the sun is starting to go down, your inflammation may start to get worse. That's why we get fevers after the doctor's office has closed. It's not poor timing on the part of sick kids. It's the level of cortisol in the body that drops at sunset and rises at sunrise. Cortisol is an anti-inflammatory that is naturally present in the body. Cortisol drops, inflammation rises. So ice is really helpful in the evening.

Stop Staring At Your Navel

Get out of yourself. Look around while you count down your second set of walkouts in physical therapy. Ask that nice man doing outer rotations how he was able to get into a t-shirt. You can't figure out how to do it and would like to know his secret. Compliment the man who is using the eight lb. weights while he does his shrugs. You'll feel much better lifting your bright pink one lb.

weights when he confides how hard it is for him to lift the eight lb. ones. And the boy in the full pillow immobilizer sling? Tell him you were there six weeks ago and encourage him to keep going, he can do it. Say hello to each of the therapists. Say hello to the receptionist who makes your appointments and prints your schedule. These people all have names. Learn them. Say thank you when you are leaving and tell them to have a good weekend or a good afternoon. During our recovery we are so focused on ourselves, we forget we live in a world full of others who would like to be recognized. We all work hard; it's nice when someone notices.

Some days you may not feel like saying a damn thing to anybody. That's okay. Try not to glare. Keep your temper and be quiet, but polite, so people don't think they did something to offend you. It's just you having a crimply, crotchety day. But keep it to 25 percent of the time. We all have bad days. Some days are going to hurt more than others. Give yourself a timeout to feel frustrated and sorry for yourself, then move on. Don't get all comfortable being spiky and closed off. You have a lot of good to share with others through a smile and a cheery hello. The person doing the pulleys next to you may have a question for you; they may have observed you and wondered how you did something? If you are open and approachable, it's easier for them to ask and learn from you or share their story with you. Shoulder surgery recovery is tough enough by itself. Don't make it any harder by building walls.

Chapter 7:

PHASE THREE

Phase Three is twelve to eighteen weeks after your surgery. Your surgeon's goals of protecting the repair, getting back full range of motion and light strengthening haven't changed. But you have! By Phase Three you'll be out of the sling and driving again. You will be wearing normal clothes and cooking your own meals. In physical therapy you'll be working on building up more strength in your arm. That's great! Be careful. Be completely present and aware of your limitations. Don't lift more than one pound with your repair arm. Be careful of any vigorous pushing or pulling with your repair arm; your repair is still healing.

I'm Fixed...Right?

You're ready to grocery shop with someone, but doing a big grocery shop by yourself is a bad idea. You're ready to run around and do errands with a friend, but a full day of errands by yourself is too much. You're ready to take a relaxing vacation, but dragging heavy suitcases by yourself is not the way to go. If you want to go on vacation, go with someone who loves you and will carry all your bags. You may carry a light purse or pull a rolling laptop bag. That's it. You're not ready to join the All-Stars in Phase Three. Your friends and family remember that you had surgery, but they're not as aware of your limitations. That's not their fault. They have moved on. They can't keep up that level of constant attention forever.

This isn't the time to feel sorry for yourself. Get fired up. Set boundaries. Say what you can and cannot do and what you will and will not do. No one is making you pick up something too heavy. No one is making you carry luggage. No one can make you do anything that is uncomfortable or that you're not ready to do. You are in charge.

Don't take your bath or shower during a busy time of day in the bathroom when everybody else in the family is trying to get ready. Choose a time when you won't feel pressured and the kids aren't buzzing around you like miniature coked up NASCAR drivers. Be relaxed and calm at all times to protect your shoulder repair.

Shopping at the grocery store is super stressful. You're not wearing a sling anymore, so people have no idea that you have an injury that you're trying to protect. They'll give you dirty looks and try to push you to move faster. Smile and take all the time you need. You can't hurry up to please them or make them feel better. You could get hurt. They have to deal with the fact that you are a slower moving human. They can take their business elsewhere or go to another check-out line if they're in that much of a rush. There are wonderful compassionate people in this world who will smile back at you and help you. And there are real jerks who will run you down with their grocery cart. Be aware and don't put yourself at the mercy of these people.

Most medical issues will make you a more compassionate person toward your fellow humanoids, but shoulder surgery will really push you in that direction. Suddenly you identify with those people who move so slowly and drive you crazy and make you late for whatever important thing you thought you should be doing. You're not a machine. You're an intricately designed creation that requires care and gentle handling. It's good to relax and enjoy your morning coffee as you lift it to your lips with a working, healing shoulder. It's even better to know there are other people in the world who can carry the trash down to the curb besides yourself.

You can go all Survivor Island when the twelve to eighteen months are done. When your surgeon says you're ready, compete with people who swim, bike, run, beat their chests and wear tribal makeup. Until then, go Tarzan while you do your shoulder exercises. If your physical therapist says that you can do extra reps, do extra reps. Put on your muscle shirt, beat your chest with your good arm and work up a sweat. Your shower will be that much more rewarding. But stay in the guidelines of rational behavior and do what your surgeon and physical therapist says. You are a surgical miracle. Eighteen months will pass and you will have a kick-ass shoulder again. So all you jackrabbits, chill out and stay with the program. This isn't a race. It's a healing.

Chapter 8:

HELPFUL TIPS

Your Armpit

Carry individually wrapped antibacterial wipes with you. There will be a moment when you're sitting down in the reception area waiting to go into physical therapy and think, "what is that awful smell?" It's you. Or rather, your armpit. You just can't get underneath there for a month or two to excavate the area. You need something with you that you can swish in there that won't disturb your repair. Anti-bacterial wipes come in individually wrapped, easily disposable packages. A baby wipe isn't strong enough to kill the odor of adult armpit bacteria. I've tried. Men: Shave the armpit of your repair arm the day before your surgery. Sounds frilly, but it works. The men are stinkier in physical therapy because of the sheer amount of toxic vegetation.

Kinesio Tape

Kinesio tape is an excellent tool in your physical therapist's bag of tricks. It helps to support surrounding muscles so you can do your exercises and work on your range of motion without so much pain. There is a specific method to putting it on. Your physical therapist can show you how to do it. You can purchase all different colors on Amazon. You can buy it in rolls and cut lengths yourself or you can buy it in pre-cut lengths. A roll costs between $10 - $15. I started using Kinesio tape in the fifth month and have used it ever since. I like the extra support.

Usually you just stick on the Kinesio tape. It adheres well and stays on for three or four showers. After a while, your skin can get irritated. There is a product by ConvaTec called AllKare. My chiropractor introduced me to it when he saw I was using the Kinesio tape. AllKare is a protective barrier wipe. You wipe it on your skin before you put on the tape. It provides a barrier skin layer under the tape to protect your skin from irritation and adhesive build-up. The wipes come in boxes of 100 individually wrapped packages for about $20.00. They work great.

Do Your Exercises Even After Your Fifth Month... Keep Going!

When you reach your fifth month, things are looking better and better. Your mobility is much improved, you're going to parties, you're back at work – you are feeling good. Normal, even. This is a challenging time because your sneaky little reptile brain is going to whisper evil thoughts in your ear. "I don't need physical therapy." "I don't need to do my exercises." "I'm fine." Don't do it! Don't cave in to the slack off monster. Your shoulder is where it's at because of hard work and diligence. This is not the time to indulge your drooling, lazy sloth. If you quit now, your shoulder can freeze up again. Keep doing those exercises three times a day. They don't have to put a crimp in your social schedule. Just keep them part of your everyday routine and keep checking off those boxes.

Don't Cancel Your Physical Therapy Appointments

Building strength is something that occurs over the entire twelve to eighteen months. It's not like you get to month nine and you magically have all your strength back. The process takes commitment. As you get busier and your schedule gets more crowded, don't neglect your physical therapy appointments. Don't cancel them. You're going to want to cancel them because you can think of a million better ways to use your time. Your physical therapist is still monitoring your range of motion and your strength. They have certain levels that they need you to attain so they can write a report for your doctor. The doctor will advise you when you are done with physical therapy. When the doctor and the physical therapist say you no longer need physical therapy, you know you are having a successful recovery.

Keep Your Incision Healthy

After four or five months your incision should be all healed and healthy. If your incision site start to sink in just a little bit, roll it around with your fingers and massage it. Don't be afraid of it. You want the skin to be smooth, supple and pliable. Sinking in can be a sign an adhesion is forming underneath. By gently moving it around you don't give the skin an opportunity to adhere to the muscle.

Baby Yourself

Probably by about the sixth or seventh month you will be released from physical therapy. You're now on your own. You'll have a check up with your surgeon just to make sure that everything is going well; but at this point, time and continued shoulder exercises are really the best healers. Time and exercise coupled with patience. Continue to use your bath chair for as long as you feel necessary. Brace yourself against the bed or a wall when you get dressed in case you lose your balance. Monitor your fatigue level.

Even during the sixth, seventh and eighth months you will get tired. You're still on the mend. Don't be so quick to fly down the driveway and get the mail. The mail will still be there when you get there. When the weather changes, there are barometric pressure changes. You're going to feel it in your shoulder. That's not a crazy wives' tale. Ask anyone who has ever had a break or sprain or surgery – they feel it in those areas. Watch out for rain, snow, ice and slippery floors in grocery stores. Be wary of elevator doors. If they start to close, get your repair arm out of the way, fast. Now that you've had shoulder surgery, you need to be aware for the rest of your life where you place your feet. You can't forestall an accident or predict someone crashing into you but you can watch where you put your feet and think about where you want to put your feet on a daily basis. You don't want to have the surgery again. Once is enough.

I always use a shopping cart to hold onto in the grocery store or in a department store like Target. Even if I'm getting just a few items, I get a cart because I don't want to slip and fall. Seven months into my shoulder repair recovery, I forgot to get a cart. After I made my purchase, I turned to leave the store. I didn't see the little girl who stepped directly in front of me. She dropped her plastic bag. I stepped on the bag, slipped sideways and tripped over the child. I did three or four hop skips and managed to stay on my feet. Too late, I remembered why I always got a cart. I mentally kicked myself for not taking my own damn advice to stay conscious of where I put my feet. I had come too far and worked too hard to be so careless. I was lucky. Thankfully, I didn't end up back in surgery. But that's how quickly it can happen – remember the cart!

Use Your Repair Wisely

Use your repaired shoulder for the things you love to do. Ask for help with everything else. Just because your shoulder is fixed doesn't mean you need to lug the world around again. Pretty much everything important gets done without your shoulder to lean on. And if it doesn't get done, it's not that important. It's a lesson in letting go of stuff you can't really control anyway. Make "working smarter, not harder" your new mantra. When you can't lift that bag of fertilizer into the back of your truck without hurting your repair, get creative. Figure out how to do stuff without hurting yourself and with the least amount of effort. Use a little common sense, good judgment and always ask for help. Maintain a good healthy shoulder.

Resuming Chores on a Regular Basis

When you resume your daily routine, chop up your chores into small bites. Schedule your grocery shopping so a family member or a neighbor can help you in with your haul. This is not the time to to hook three bags on your good arm and attempt to hold the screen door open with your rear end as you puff up the stairs into the kitchen. Buy smaller amounts and shop more often. Or order online and have it delivered. Don't reach overhead for dishes and holiday decorations stored in the attic. Be reasonable. Don't end up back in Phase One out of pure stubbornness.

If you must vacuum, use your good arm and do a small area. Sit down and see how your shoulder feels. It may take longer. So what? So many of us are overachievers. Sweeping and vacuuming use your whole shoulder. Ask your physical therapist their opinion before you try it on your own. They know your capabilities. Try short intervals and wait twenty-four hours to see how it affects your repair. A sweeping motion makes my shoulder feel sore. I've tried so many vacuums looking for one that is light and easy on my shoulder. My favorite one so far is the Hoover Corded Cyclonic Stick Vacuum, SH20030. It sells for around $80 and is delivered free to your door with Amazon Prime.

For those moments when you must dust bust or go mad because tumbleweeds of dog hair mixed with old food crumbs keep drifting by, the lightweight Black and Decker BDH 2000PL MAX Lithium Pivot Vacuum, 20 volt with compact charging station is the way to go. I have never been so infatuated with a hand vac. Its nozzle pivots for all those hard to reach places, it has amazingly strong suction and the lithium ion batteries give it long lasting power. I almost feel like I need to buy it dinner when I'm done. It's extravagant at $70, but worth every penny.

Save your enthusiasm and "git 'er done" attitude for your range of motion and strength exercises. These exercises will help you so much more in the long run than a dust bunny free house. There's a saying: "how nice to do nothing and then rest afterward."

Going Out on the Town Before You're Ready

You may not feel like going out to dinner until you're in Phase Two and maybe not even until halfway through that. That's what take-out is for. That's what friends, who bring over those amazingly good home-cooked meals because they love you, are for. Protect your repair.

When you finally feel like going out to dinner, it's an entire process in itself. Take at least 45 minutes to bathe. Take another 30 minutes to dress. Make sure you take your pain medication and you have ample time to get out to the car. In the first few months of recovery, spontaneity goes out the window. You can't be spontaneous when you're in a sling. It's hard to zip through a shower when you move like Yertle the Turtle. Sometimes you just feel so drained, you don't feel like putting on your eyes or your lips. You don't feel like washing your hair so it's a pokey up, greasy, nasty bird's nest mess on top of your head.

The restaurants will be waiting for you. The movie theaters and vacations will be waiting for you. This is the time to watch the grass grow. Waiting while your shoulder heals and you dutifully do your exercises is about as interesting as watching paint dry. It's not a fun time, but it can be a fruitful time. Take up meditation. Sit and talk with friends you haven't talked to for a long time because you were too busy before surgery. Right now you have all the time in the world. It's intriguing to be the one sitting down while everybody else dashes around. You're the calm eye in the storm. You'll re-enter the storm at some point, but not yet. You'll realize when your child's dish of lasagna lands on the carpet, you can't do anything about it. Either somebody will clean it up or the dog will eat it. Relax and take a nap.

HALT for Shoulder Surgery Recovery

Borrowing a concept from twelve-step groups, HALT stands for Hungry, Angry, Lonely and Tired. These are times to be aware and pay attention. Any one of these four states can influence how you care for yourself and your shoulder repair. If I am feeling any of these four, it's a warning signal for me to watch out.

Hunger is obvious. Have those raisins, crackers, granola bars, cheese sticks and other snack items available. While you are in the sling, make sure you can open these items with one hand or ask someone to help you. Get the food into you. Hunger can lead to dizziness and falling. Hunger can also lead to fuzzy thinking and maybe trying to lift or do something that could damage your repair.

Anger is going to happen. Be aware when it happens. You're going to get irritated at the people trying to help you. You're going to be frustrated at yourself when you can't make your recovery go faster. You're going to get angry at people you don't even know because you're in pain. When you get angry you start to do stupid things like kicking the kitchen trash can with your foot. Hard. You can break a toe that way. I did. I was blowing off steam because I was angry. Somebody didn't do something I needed them to do. I felt helpless, vulnerable and plain old mad. Hurting myself didn't make the situation better. Be careful. Don't yank the dryer door open with your repair arm while thinking angry thoughts. That extra energy output could hurt you!

Lonely isn't so obvious. It creeps up on you. It's lonely when you've had shoulder surgery. You're by yourself in a recliner, staring at the wall feeling blue. You think nobody cares. You don't want to bother anybody. Make the effort to dial the phone and call a friend. Share your feelings. Say "Hi. Got a minute? I need someone to talk to and I was wondering what's happening in your life?" Texting a friend is good, but hearing their voice is better.

Chatting with a friend will lift your spirits and get you out of yourself.

Tired is something we have to be on guard against at all times. Shoulder surgery knocks the stuffing out of us. We need to rest and sleep a lot. Our body is busy growing cells and re-attaching a tendon to a bone. You're giving birth to a baby shoulder. Be tuned into your body. It will give you warning signals when you're overdoing it. It will let you know when you're fatiguing your muscles. Your body knows when you're about to go too far and get so tired you burst into tears or yell at the person next to you.

Chapter 9:

PHASE FOUR AND BEYOND

Phase Four is roughly eighteen to twenty-eight weeks after your surgery. Most hospitals and orthopedic surgeons follow a similar protocol: protect your repair, get back your full range of motion, get back your full strength and get you back to your normal activities. You still have to be careful to avoid using your arm in a vigorous manner. You still have to hold off on lifting heavy stuff with your repair arm.

Try to distribute weight evenly between your hands when carrying items. Don't attempt to hold too much in one hand. Keep your other arm in shape as well. Do your exercises on both sides to have the best range of motion and strength in each arm. Remember to continue to do your exercises; it's the best way to keep your repair in shape and keep you in tune with your body. Ice is your best buddy if you overdo. Keep your cold packs ready to go in the freezer.

Your doctor and your physical therapist are there to give you specific instructions to help you return to your favorite sports and activities. Keep listening to that shoulder. You need to regain full range of motion, have full strength and have no pain or swelling before you go back to most sports. If you want to return to weight training, you need to check with your doctor for appropriate advice and guidelines.

Shoulder surgery helped me play my guitar again. It taught me how to move through my fear of pain and loss of control. I put my foot on the brakes and began to listen to my body. I discovered a new-found knowledge and appreciation of physical therapy. Physical therapy is your lifeline to becoming a strong, active person again after you have taken the steps to repair your shoulder with surgery.

I approach life differently now. People swirl around me, running to and fro, intent on where they're headed. As for me and my shoulder, we're content to watch. We're a team now. Exercises are a permanent part of our life, not an option. And we steadfastly refuse to do any action that would jeopardize the repair. The repair is our number one priority.

I don't expect you to wrap yourself in bubble wrap. Just try not to do anything stupid on purpose or think you're done when your shoulder's only half-baked and not ready to come out of the oven yet. Your doctor and your physical therapist know what they're doing. Listen to them.

Now's the time to catch up on all the television series you've heard about but never had the time to watch. Amaze your friends with how chill and hip you are from all the documentaries you're watching. And if anybody busts your chops about how long your recovery is taking, just smile and walk on by. No one's gonna rain on your recovery parade – keep marching front and center. Eyes on the prize, baby, eyes on the prize...a fully healed, fully functional shoulder.

If you or someone you know decides to have shoulder surgery in the future, remember the 3 P's:

* **Preparation**
* **Practice**
* **Physical Therapy**

Take charge of the process. You can do this. Do your prep, do your practice and do your physical therapy. Together, they are your key to a successful, stress-free recovery.

APPENDIX

Teaching Textbooks: teachingtextbooks.com
Super Teacher Worksheets: superteacherworksheets.com
Time4Learning: time4learning.com
Scholastic Worksheets: scholastic.com

GrubHub: grubhub.com
Blue Apron: blueapron.com
Plated: plated.com
HelloFresh: hellofresh.com
Home Chef: homechef.com
PeachDish: peachdish.com
Schwan's Grocery/Delivery: schwans.com
Prime Pantry: amazon.com

Netflix: netflix.com
ROKU: roku.com
Gaiam TV: gaiamtv.com

ShoulderShirts: Etsy/Amazon
DressWithEase: Etsy/Amazon
BlossomBreeze: Amazon

APPENDIX (continued)

Self-Wipe Toilet Aid: RehabMart.com

Amazon.com:

Comfort Choice Women's Posture Support Soft Cup Bra
Glamorise Magic Lift Wireless Front Hook Posture Bra
Wacoal Women's Plus-Size Full Figure Red Carpet
Strapless Bra

SOFSOLE Performance Stretch Laces:
sofsole.com
HICKIES for shoes: hickies.com

Shoulder Cryo Cuff: amazon.com
ALEVA Bamboo Baby Wipes: amazon.com
CAREX Quick-Lock Raised Toilet Seat:
walmart.com
AquaSense Adjustable Bath Chair w/Non-Slip Seat &
Backrest: walgreens.com

APPENDIX (continued)

WrightStuff.biz
- rocker knives
- jar, bag and bottle openers
- non-slip mats
- Fiskar scissors
- soap holders
- leather weights
- 2-handled coffee cups

Amazon.com
- Sunshine Pillow Chiropractic Neck Support Pillow
- Homedics OT-LUM Therapy Lumbar Cushion Support Pillow
- Coccyx Gel Seat Cushion w/Fleece Top
- Jobri Spine Reliever Bed Wedge
- Jobri Spine Reliever Leg Wedge
- Marpac DOHM-DS Natural White Noise Sound Machine
- Shoulder Abduction Sling with Pillow
- Kinesio Tape
- AllKare by ConvaTec -- protective barrier wipe for use with Kinesio Tape

APPENDIX (continued)

- Colpac Cold Therapy Packs
- Comfort Bath Personal Cleansing Ultra-Thick Disposable Washcloths
- Thera-Med Reusable Cold Packs
- Hoover Corded Cyclonic Stick Vacuum, SH20030
- Black and Decker BDH 2000PL MAX Lithium Pivot Vacuum, 20 Volt

Special appreciation to:

Martin Knee and Sports Medicine
Out Patient Physical Therapy at CHI St. Vincent
The Massachusetts General Hospital Sports Medicine and Orthopedic Group
Brigham and Women's Hospital, Inc. Department of Rehabilitation Services

You provided my addled and pain-confused brain with a constant inflow of information. With your help I muddled through each day and sought to understand what the hell was going on with my shoulder during all phases of my recovery. You gave me a road map. I followed it and arrived at my destination with my arm intact. Thank you.

There's always something new around the corner...

Stay in touch with the author via:

Email: annetalmage@gmail.com

Website: http://annetalmage.wix.com/annetalmagecooksey

Instagram: https://instagram.com/annetalmagecooksey

Facebook: Anne Talmage Cooksey

Twitter: https://twitter.com/talmageanne

If you liked ***Shoulder Surgery Recovery***, please post a review at Amazon and let your friends know about the book.

Made in the USA
Middletown, DE
07 May 2016